THE GENERAL PRACTICE MANUALS

(OTHER TITLES IN PREPARATION)

PICTORIAL HANDBOOK

of

FRACTURE TREATMENT

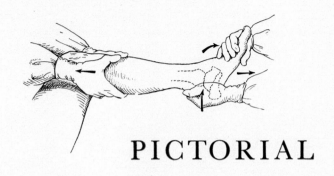

PICTORIAL

Illustrated by

HAROLD LAUFMAN, M.D., F.A.C.S.

Department of Surgery, Northwestern University Medical School

THIRD EDITION

HANDBOOK *of*

Fracture Treatment

EDWARD L. COMPERE, M.D., F.A.C.S.

Professor and Chairman of Department of Bone and Joint Surgery, Northwestern University Medical School; Chairman, Departments of Orthopaedic Surgery, Wesley Memorial and Children's Memorial Hospitals; Consultant in Orthopaedics, Chicago Memorial and Henrotin Hospitals; Medical Adviser and Director, Rehabilitation Center of The Liberty Mutual Insurance Company, Chicago

SAM W. BANKS, M.D., F.A.C.S.

Associate Professor of Surgery, Northwestern University Medical School; Attending Orthopaedic Surgeon, Chicago Memorial, Woodlawn and Hines Veterans Hospitals, Chicago

Revised with the Assistance of

CLINTON L. COMPERE, M.D., F.A.C.S.

Assistant Professor of Surgery, Northwestern University Medical School; Attending Orthopaedic Surgeon, Wesley Memorial Hospital; Consultant in Orthopaedic Surgery, Augustana Hospital; Senior Consultant, Veterans Administration, Chicago

CHICAGO, ILL.

THE YEAR BOOK PUBLISHERS · INC.

First Edition, June, 1943
Revised and Reprinted, December, 1943
Second Edition, August, 1947
Reprinted, January, 1949
Reprinted, July, 1951
Third Edition, August, 1952
Reprinted, November, 1953

PRINTED IN U. S. A.

Preface to Third Edition

ALTHOUGH THERE have been several reprintings of the *Pictorial Handbook of Fracture Treatment* during the past four years, this is the first complete revision since August of 1947.

The new edition of the *Standard Nomenclature of Diseases and Operations,* prepared by the American Medical Association, does not accept the terms "simple" and "compound" to denote "closed" and "open" fractures. The term "simple fracture" has been very confusing to lay people and some insurance company representatives. Adjusters for insurance companies providing coverage for patients insured against traumatic injuries have been inclined to complain that charges made for the care of very difficult fractures listed as "simple" were too high. Similarly, the word "compound" connotes nothing of significance. We use the terms *open* and *closed* instead of "compound" and "simple" throughout this revised edition.

During and following World War II, improvements in the techniques of the care of fractures have been described by various orthopedic and traumatic surgeons. Those new techniques which we have found to be useful are described in this revision.

During the past few years we have become more certain about the indications for the use of the intramedullary nail, the internal fixation of fractures of the neck of the femur, arthroplasty of the hip, or prosthetic replacements for the necrotic head of the femur. The importance of maintaining continuous contact between fracture surfaces by the physiologic pressure forces of the muscles surrounding the fractured bone fragments has become more generally acknowledged during the past few years. Absorption of the ends of the fracture fragments results in slight shortening of these fragments. If immobilization has been by rigid metal plates, the ends of the fragments will lose contact with each other, the compression force between the fragments is lost and nonunions are more likely to occur. Methods of treatment which will utilize this principle of contact compression have been described in this edition.

Chapters I, XIV and XXIV, dealing with fracture pathology, aseptic necrosis of bone and fractures of the hip, have been rewritten, and many changes have been made in other chapters of this book. Many of the diagrammatic illustrations have been redrawn and several new drawings have been added. New roentgenograms and photographs which help to explain problems of treatment of fractures will be found in each of several chapters. Although we have tried to avoid increasing the size of the book, it has been impossible to include this new material without adding a few pages. This edition of the *Pictorial Handbook of Fracture Treatment* is offered in the hope that it will be of real help to medical students and to the physician in general practice who wishes to provide, for his patients who have suffered fracture or dislocation injuries, the very best orthopedic care.

—EDWARD L. COMPERE.
—SAM W. BANKS.
—CLINTON L. COMPERE.

Preface to First Edition

SOME FIVE THOUSAND years ago an Egyptian scribe lamented that the world was rapidly becoming demoralized, children no longer obeyed their parents and everyone was trying to write a book! There are many who believe that this situation prevails today, and some may ask, "Why *another* book on fractures?"

Indeed it is true that during the last decade the subject of fractures has been in high favor. Many volumes, some of them excellent, have been published in the British Isles and Continental Europe, as well as in the United States of America, and any physician who undertakes to treat a large number of injuries to the bones and joints should consider at least one of them indispensable for reference. The best of them, however, are large and encyclopedic. For the doctor in general practice, they may seem formidable. The material is too lengthy for the limited time that he has to give to this particular part of his practice; he becomes lost in the maze of details and bewildered in the attempt to decide which of several methods he should use. The medical student, intern or hospital resident may likewise be discouraged.

Smaller textbooks on fractures have appeared, but for the most part they have failed to provide the mental or visual picture of the actual steps required to reduce, immobilize and provide intelligent after-care for each of the more common fractures or dislocation injuries. There does exist, then, at this time, an

9

especial need for a text on fractures, a text which presents concisely but adequately the procedures indicated in treatment of the more common injuries, and to this end the authors of this volume have devoted their efforts.

Industry, the automobile and, more recently, mechanized warfare have increased tremendously the incidence of fractures, dislocations and other injuries to the skeletal system of the human body. Multiple fractures are common. Severe trauma to the soft tissues may accompany and complicate the fractures or dislocations. Compound fractures are more common today than at any previous time. Wise and skilful management of these injuries may mean the difference between complete recovery and lifelong invalidism.

In large hospitals where there are physicians trained in the disciplines of fracture therapy, the injury cases are well managed. But fractures and other injuries to the spine and extremities have no predilection for urban locale. They occur in every village and countryside, and the physician in the small town or rural area must treat them. He may not be interested primarily in fractures, but there is no orthopedic surgeon across the hall to whom he may refer the case. These are the men for whom this book has been prepared—the conscientious, overworked country doctors and general practitioners, and the medical students who will be treating the injuries of tomorrow.

In preparing this book, the authors have avoided presentation of several different methods of management for each type of injury. It is better to know one method well and to be able to apply it with assurance and skill than to have a less thorough knowledge of several techniques. Therefore the simplest principles and methods by which the authors themselves have been able consistently to obtain a satisfactory end-result have been presented, and no references are made to certain methods of fracture management which have proved successful in the hands of other physicians. Little reference has been made to the wide assortment of gadgets and automatic reducing devices, because they are seldom available to the general practitioner. On the other hand, we have tried to present with especial clarity the technique of skeletal traction and the use of internal fixation for certain fractures, since these should be a part of the armamentarium of any doctor who undertakes the care of bone and joint injuries.

We have used freely the excellent reference texts by many of our colleagues and preceptors on the subject of fractures and dislocations and are greatly indebted to Roger Anderson, Lorenz Boehler, Willis Campbell, Albert Key and Earl Conwell, Paul Magnuson, Charles Scudder, Kellogg Speed and Reginald Watson-Jones. We wish to express appreciation to those who have given so generously of their time in helping with various phases of this manual, to Jean Nolan for editorial assistance and especially to Dr. Harold Laufman, artist and surgeon, whose unique skill in preparing the drawings has made possible the visual presentation of the methods described. To the Department of Surgery of the University of Chicago, we are grateful for having been granted permission to use the roentgenograms of patients treated in the University Clinics.

—Edward L. Compere.

—Sam W. Banks.

Table of Contents

PART III. *Fractures and Dislocations of the Lower Limbs*

PART IV. *Fractures and Dislocations of the Trunk*

PART V. *The Face and Skull*

PART I

General Considerations of
Treatment of Fractures and Dislocations

CHAPTER I

Fracture Pathology

THE classic definition of fracture is "a break in the continuity of bone." For many years those who were concerned about accuracy of terminology have objected to some of the terms used to describe certain fractures. In the 1951 edition of the *Standard Nomenclature of Diseases and Operations* published by the American Medical Association, all fractures in which the fractured bone end protrudes through the skin, or an object penetrates the skin and subcutaneous tissue to the site of the break, are called *open* fractures instead of "compound" fractures. Similarly, when there is no communication between the skin and the fracture, or between one of the body cavities and the fracture, the term *closed* is used instead of "simple." The old classifications "compound" and "simple" are no longer used. It is hoped that all physicians and surgeons working with orthopedic and traumatic conditions will assist in popularizing the new terminology.

All *open* fractures are potentially infected. They require emergency care. In either a closed or an open fracture the ends of the fragments may be separated *(displaced)*, driven into each other *(impacted)* or shattered into pieces *(comminuted)*.

The forces which produce fractures may be direct or indirect. Direct violence results from impact, as when a pedestrian is struck by an automobile or a passenger is thrown forcibly against the dashboard or the top of the car. *Direct* fractures are frequently open and comminuted. *Indirect* forces produced by torsion, traction or leverage frequently result in oblique, linear and avulsion fractures.

Fractures may be grouped according to the age of the patient. Those which occur before or at the time of delivery of an infant are known as *birth fractures*. Incomplete fractures, common in children, have been designated *greenstick fractures*. Separation of an epiphysis from the shaft of a bone at the plane of cleavage occupied by the growth cartilage plate is sometimes designated *slipped epiphysis,* but may be classed as an epiphyseal fracture. This is a rare injury in young children and is most common during puberty.

Fracture fragments may penetrate the peritoneal cavity, the thorax, or may injure such organs as the liver, the kidney, the spleen or the lungs. Fractures of the spine may produce severe trauma to the spinal cord, including partial or complete transection.

Bone is a living tissue and requires an adequate blood supply. Fractures disrupt blood vessels. The amount of hemorrhage will vary according to the location of the fracture with respect to the major nutrient blood vessels and to the degree of trauma which accompanies a break of the bone. The muscles, ligaments, nerves and other soft tissues may be severely traumatized and occasionally may be interposed in the fracture. This may defeat attempts at reduction and is one cause of nonunion. In a closed fracture the blood is usually confined to the region of the fracture and forms a hematoma. With greater injury to the soft tissues at the site of fracture, the blood may extravasate, producing marked discoloration of the skin. Also, blood may migrate along the planes of the intermuscular septa or directly beneath the skin, in directions determined by the force of gravity, to locations distal to the site of fracture and the origin of the bleeding. The presence of large amounts of blood in the soft tissues may cause a febrile reaction which results from the disintegration and absorption of blood protein substances. Pain is produced by motion or disturbance of the injured part. It gives rise to protective muscle spasm, and the cramp-like spasm may cause further pain. The pain and spasm are minimized or relieved by adequate immobilization.

CHAPTER II

Fracture Healing

THE repair of a defect in any tissue is initiated by an ingrowth of fibroblasts, resulting in a scarlike union by granulation tissue. The healing processes of a closed fracture consist of the following stages.

1. Formation of a clot in the hematoma around the ends of the fragments.
2. Invasion of the clot by fibroblasts and capillaries, with gradual transformation into a mass of immature connective tissue.
3. The deposition of calcium in the connective tissue, forming what is recognized both roentgenographically and microscopically as callus.
4. Absorption of devitalized bone from the ends of the fracture fragments.
5. Transition of the callus into osteoid tissue and deposition of bone.
6. Consolidation and reorganization of the newly formed bone, with decrease in the size of the bony mass.

If the periosteum is not widely torn at the time of fracture, it will confine the hematoma locally, and the subsequent callus will be smoothly outlined in the roentgenogram. If the hematoma escapes, as it does if the fracture is open or if an open operation is performed, the normal process of fracture healing may be hindered. Since the hematoma plays an important role in the first stages of fracture healing, it should be preserved whenever possible.

Too much traction with separation of the fracture fragments and plating of the fracture with the ends of the fragments not in good contact with each other are common causes for delayed or nonunion. Immobilization of the fracture by means of an intramedullary rod, a slotted plate or a plaster of paris cast will permit the continued maintenance of physiologic compression between the fracture surfaces. This compression is physiologic when it is produced by the tonus present in the muscles which surround and span the fracture. Fracture healing will be hastened and the incidence of delayed or nonunion greatly reduced if this principle of mild compression is fully understood and utilized.

The stimulus for the repair of a fracture is greatest during the first few days after the injury. If accurate reduction and adequate fixation are delayed for several weeks most of this *osteogenetic push* will have been lost. Separate or detached bone fragments, including large tubular segments of major long bones, are very likely to undergo aseptic necrosis and to cause union to be long delayed.

Final healing of the fracture is achieved when the medullary canal has been restored by absorption of the centrally formed bone and replacement with fine trabeculae—a process known as *tubulation*. For most major bones, the complete restoration of structural strength in continuity and tubulation, with the reappearance of fat and marrow cells, requires about one year.

CHAPTER III

The Diagnosis of Fracture

A HISTORY of an injury, which may be that of a fall, a torsion strain, an automobile accident, a blow from a blunt object, the blast of a shell or direct impact from a bullet or a bomb fragment, calls for an adequate examination to determine the presence or absence of a fracture or fractures. The characteristic complaints of a patient who has sustained a fracture are localized pain and inability to use the injured part or extremity.

The complete loss of continuity of any major bone produces such interference with function of the extremity that diagnosis of fracture may be made on minimal examination. Incomplete or impacted fractures may be accompanied by relatively little pain or local changes, making the diagnosis difficult to confirm, even with good roentgenograms.

The PHYSICAL FINDINGS which suggest the possibility of a broken bone are: (1) local swelling; (2) tenderness; (3) deformity; (4) false motion; (5) crepitation; (6) ecchymosis, and (7) muscle spasm.

1. *Local swelling* may not be demonstrable if the fractured bone lies deep within the soft parts, as the neck of the femur or a vertebral body, or if the fragments are well impacted.

2. *Bone tenderness* may be relatively minimal if the fracture

is impacted, but its presence should always suggest the possibility of a fracture.

3. *Deformity* may include angulation of a long bone (as of the humerus, femur or clavicle), shortening (due to over-riding or impaction of fragments) or mal-alignment of a joint.

4. *False motion* will be demonstrable if the fracture is complete and not impacted. Attempts to demonstrate this should be made with caution because of the possibility of creating further injury to nerves, blood vessels or other soft parts.

5. The crunching together of the ends of the fragments produces a palpable crackling or crunching sensation known as *crepitation*.

6. The presence of discoloration of the skin, due to hemorrhage which has extravasated into the subcutaneous tissues, is known as *ecchymosis*.

7. *Muscle spasm* is a protective phenomenon in which the muscles become markedly contracted in an attempt to splint the fracture fragments and prevent motion between them. Spasm is increased by manual attempts to move the extremity or to produce motion at the site of the fracture.

Confirmation of the presence of a fracture is obtained by roentgenograms. X-rays taken for this purpose should always include at least two planes, the anteroposterior and a lateral view. Certain fractures are best demonstrated by taking oblique roentgenograms. Multiple plane roentgenograms are helpful not only in making the diagnosis and in accurately determining the position of the fragments, but also by affording visual aid to the surgeon in manipulating and reducing the fracture. Fluoroscopy, at least by those who are not fully trained in roentgen techniques, is unreliable either for the diagnosis of fractures or for confirmation of the reduction and may be very deceptive.

CHAPTER IV

Emergency Treatment
of Fractures

Every fracture of a major bone should be splinted before the patient is moved from the site of the injury. Fractures that are confined solely to the small bones of the hand or foot may not require this precaution, but if the injury is obviously severe, involving the spine or one of the long bones, such as the shaft of the femur, the tibia or the humerus, or if the patient is unconscious, much additional trauma may be inflicted by careless, ignorant or indifferent handling (Fig. 1). For a leg fracture, the use of a Thomas splint, with traction applied to the foot or shoe of the victim, will reduce the danger of inflicting additional injury to soft parts and of opening a closed fracture, or further contaminating the open fracture wound (Fig. 2).

Pain is best alleviated by an adequate dose of morphine and immediate immobilization. For an adult the dose should be $\frac{1}{4}$ gr.; for a teen-age child, $\frac{1}{8}$ gr.; in a younger child, it may be omitted. *Narcotics should be withheld if there is evidence of cerebral concussion.* The first aid team should make no attempt to sterilize the wound. The use of strong antiseptics like iodine should not be permitted. Open wounds should be covered with a

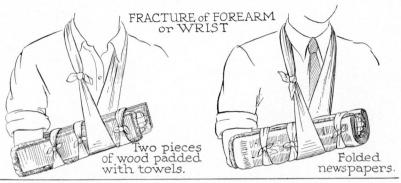

FRACTURE of FOREARM
or WRIST

Two pieces
of wood padded
with towels.

Folded
newspapers.

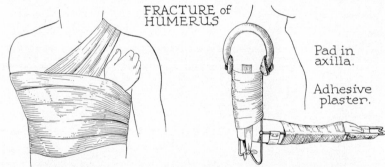

FRACTURE of
HUMERUS

Pad in
axilla.

Adhesive
plaster.

Arm bandaged to body,
pad in axilla

Modified Thomas splint for
compound fractures or for
distant transportation.

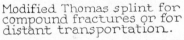

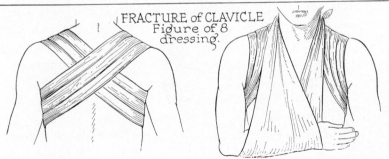

FRACTURE of CLAVICLE
Figure of 8
dressing.

FIG. 1.—First aid splinting of fractures of the upper extremity.

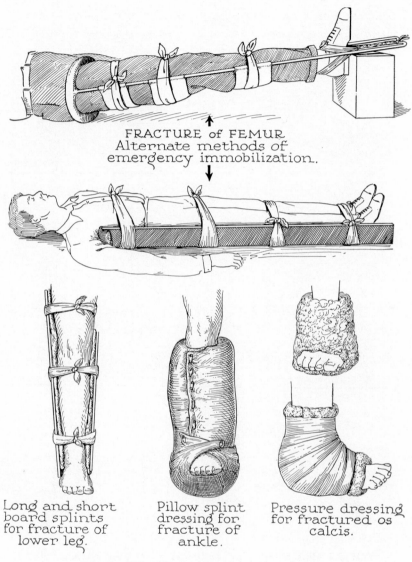

FRACTURE of FEMUR
Alternate methods of
emergency immobilization.

Long and short board splints for fracture of lower leg.

Pillow splint dressing for fracture of ankle.

Pressure dressing for fractured os calcis.

FIG. 2.—First aid splinting of the lower extremity.

clean cloth or sterile pressure dressing. The patient must be kept warm and transported, with minimal delay, to a hospital. If several hours may intervene before definitive treatment can be given,

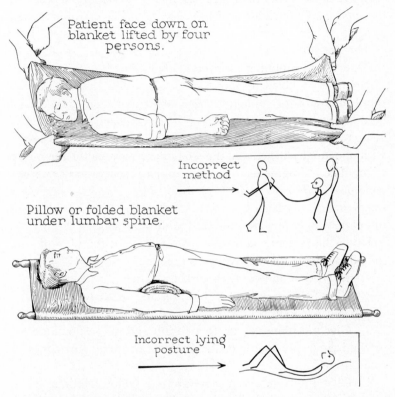

Patient face down on blanket lifted by four persons.

Incorrect method

Pillow or folded blanket under lumbar spine.

Incorrect lying posture

Fig. 3.—Correct method of lifting and transporting a patient who has suffered an injury to the spine.

a single injection of 600,000 units of penicillin should be administered as soon as possible.

PRIMARY SHOCK may be combated by morphine, the control of hemorrhage by pressure dressings and replacement of lost blood. A tourniquet may be necessary to control massive bleeding, but its prolonged use has resulted too often in gangrene and the subsequent loss of an arm or leg.

Except for the control of hemorrhage, emergency treatment rarely requires haste. Breath-taking rides in speeding ambulances are more likely to result in death than to aid in the preservation of life.

The patient should be carried to a hospital on a stretcher or transported by ambulance or automobile (Fig. 3). Never should a patient be doubled up into the back seat of a car. A compression fracture of the spine may become a transection of the spinal cord, or a closed fracture may become an open fracture. The common practice of lifting a patient under the arms and knees, with the thighs flexed on the abdomen, may cause the sharp edges of bone fragments to lacerate major blood vessels or nerves. *Ambulance drivers should be instructed to proceed slowly over rough streets and around corners.* Precaution to avoid jolting of the patient may prevent pain and additional shock.

Upon the patient's admission to the hospital the plan of care should consist of the following routine:

1. Inspection and evaluation of the patient.

2. Check the pulse and respiration and, if there are signs of shock, check blood pressure.

3. Give morphine, $\frac{1}{4}$ gr. to an adult and proportionate doses to children (morphine is contraindicated if there is evidence of brain injury).

4. Give fluids intravenously—normal saline solution, blood plasma, serum or whole blood—to relieve shock.

5. Apply splint or other immobilization to the fracture.

6. Obtain roentgenograms after shock is controlled.

CHAPTER V

Anesthesia

REDUCTION of fractures by manipulation should be carried out under anesthesia—general, regional or local.

The splints which were applied as a first aid measure or following previous attempts at reduction should not be removed until the anesthesia (either regional or general) is complete. The patient will be less apprehensive, unnecessary pain will be prevented, and the fracture will be protected from trauma which might occur during an excitement stage of general anesthesia.

General anesthesia may be induced by ether, nitrous oxide, ethylene, cyclopropane or the increasingly popular general anesthetic administered intravenously, Pentothal sodium. For those who are not thoroughly trained in the techniques of general anesthesia, ether is the safest. Anesthetic gases, such as those listed, should be administered only by physicians or nurses who are fully aware of their dangers and adequately equipped with the materials necessary for counteracting the bad effects when they do appear. Muscular relaxation is more readily obtained with ether than with anesthetic gases.

Intravenous anesthesia by means of Pentothal sodium has been eminently satisfactory. Only occasionally does this method fail to effect complete muscular relaxation. Pentothal sodium also simplifies the handling of a patient during the manipulation of fractures under fluoroscopic control. Its use is contraindicated in patients who have low blood pressure, serious organic cardiac disease or renal disease, and it is considered less safe for young children than for adults. (Oxygen should be readily available when Pentothal is used.)

Regional anesthesia is obtained by procaine block of the major nerves which supply an entire extremity or a segment of an arm or leg. This form of anesthesia may be used when general or local anesthesia is contraindicated. Its success depends on the skill and experience of the physician in locating the nerves with the point of the needle. Its advantages over general anesthesia are that the patient does not lose consciousness and that there is less danger of upper respiratory complications or aspiration pneumonia. The most commonly used regional anesthesia is that known as spinal, in which procaine is injected into the subarachnoid space, producing complete flaccid paralysis of the lower extremities. Other forms of regional anesthesia obtainable with procaine are:

1. Upper extremity. Inject the brachial plexus at a point just above the midportion of the clavicle. Avoid the subclavian artery.

2. Forearm and hand. Inject procaine in a ring around the arm just below the elbow and around the median and ulnar nerves.

3. Lower extremity. Inject the sciatic nerve where it emerges from the sciatic notch and the femoral nerve where it enters the thigh below the inguinal ligament.

4. Finger or toe. Infiltrate procaine around the base of the part and inject the digital nerves. Epinephrine should not be used in procaine for circular infiltration of fingers or toes.

Local anesthesia is by far the safest and most practical for the management of certain fractures of the extremities and is definitely to be preferred when the fracture management is undertaken in the physician's office which often is not equipped for the safe administration of inhalation or intravenous anesthesia. Local anesthesia should be used in all cases in which both general and

the position secure. Pins placed through the bone above and below the site of fracture may be incorporated in the plaster dressing, or they may be connected by special external steel bars without the use of plaster, thus maintaining both traction and reduction while permitting ambulation.

When the operator prefers continuous traction without rigid immobilization, it may be obtained by adhesive or skeletal traction, with the patient in bed and the extremity on a Thomas or

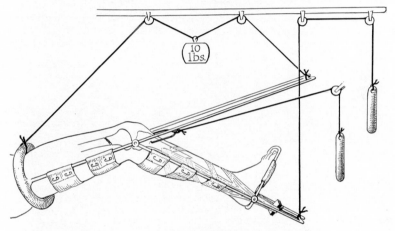

Fig. 5.—Balanced traction in a Thomas splint. The Pierson attachment permits motion of the knee while the fracture is healing.

Braun splint (Fig. 5). Care should be taken to relax the adjacent joint structures and, if possible, to maintain motion in them. Lessons learned in the British Isles and in other theaters during the recent war have emphasized the advantages of maximal immobilization of the fracture with minimal immobilization of the patient.

Russell traction is the most effective temporary or initial treatment of fractures of the proximal end or neck of the femur. It simplifies nursing care, the patient is usually quite comfortable, and adequate reduction for subsequent internal fixation is often obtained.

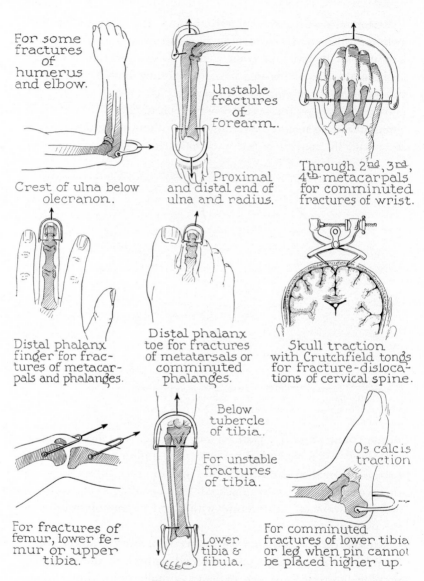

For some fractures of humerus and elbow.

Crest of ulna below olecranon.

Unstable fractures of forearm.

Proximal and distal end of ulna and radius.

Through 2nd, 3rd, 4th metacarpals for comminuted fractures of wrist.

Distal phalanx finger for fractures of metacarpals and phalanges.

Distal phalanx toe for fractures of metatarsals or comminuted phalanges.

Skull traction with Crutchfield tongs for fracture-dislocations of cervical spine.

For fractures of femur, lower femur or upper tibia.

Below tubercle of tibia.

For unstable fractures of tibia.

Lower tibia & fibula.

Os calcis traction

For comminuted fractures of lower tibia or leg when pin cannot be placed higher up.

Fig. 6.—Skeletal traction.

36

Restoration to normal position, length and alignment is the goal in reduction of every fracture. The limb or the spine should have normal function when the surgeon has completed his job and the fracture has healed. The fracture surgeon should strive for both anatomic and physiologic perfection, even though he knows that such perfection is rarely possible. To determine whether a reduction is satisfactory, the following factors should be considered:

1. Restoration of length.
2. Realignment of bone and adjacent joints.
3. Correction of rotational displacement.
4. Apposition of fragment ends, sufficient to assure healing.
5. Acceptable reduction verified by roentgenograms.

Completely accurate re-position of the fracture surfaces of fragments is not always necessary for an excellent functional result.

TABLE 1.—SITES OF INSERTION OF PINS FOR SKELETAL TRACTION

SITE FOR INSERTION	REASON FOR TRACTION	
	Fracture of Bone	Injury to Joint
Olecranon	Humerus	Shoulder and elbow
Lower radius and ulna	Shaft of radius and ulna	Elbow
Metacarpals	Lower end of radius	Wrist
Phalanges (fingers)	Metacarpals, phalanges	Interphalangeal
Greater trochanter	Central fracture of acetabulum	Hip
Lower femur	Middle or upper third of femur	Hip
Upper tibial crest	Condyles or shaft of femur	Knee
Lower tibial crest	Shaft of tibia	Knee
Os calcis	Shaft of tibia or femur (if condition of skin does not allow use of lower femur or upper tibia)	Ankle
Phalanges (toes)	Metatarsals, phalanges	Midtarsal; interphalangeal

When the fracture extends into a joint, exact anatomic reduction, however, is essential for the restoration of good function and for the prevention of traumatic arthritis. Frequent roentgenographic examinations should be made. Fluoroscopic examination is inadequate, and its routine use exposes the operator to excessive irradiation. The roentgenogram more accurately portrays detail.

When using skeletal traction the pins or wires should not be passed through tendons or close to articular surfaces (Fig. 6), because any foreign body, even though inert, may produce mechanical irritation that will result in joint inflammation or tenosynovitis with adhesions and thereby cause loss of function. Table 1 shows the sites for insertion of pins for certain fractures of bones and injuries to joints.

CHAPTER VII

Immobilization of Fractures

FROM the standpoint of obtaining satisfactory results in the management of fractures, adequate immobilization is next in importance to accurate reduction. Lack of adequate immobilization, or the discontinuance of immobilization before there is good evidence of union of the fracture as demonstrated roentgenologically, constitutes the foremost cause of all non-unions.

Circumspect planning is required in deciding which method to use. The ever-present economic problem should not be overlooked, and if adequate immobilization can be obtained by means which will permit the patient to be ambulatory and to leave the hospital before he is financially embarrassed, both patient and physician will benefit thereby. Ambulation, when possible, will aid in establishing early functional activity. The wastage of tissues from atrophy of disuse can be reduced by making possible maximum function of the injured extremity and of the body as a whole. This activity stimulates repair of the bone, is beneficial to the circulation in general, prevents wastage and weakening of muscles and minimizes the atrophy of the joint structures, with its attendant loss of function. Ambulatory patients rarely become psychologic invalids and are much

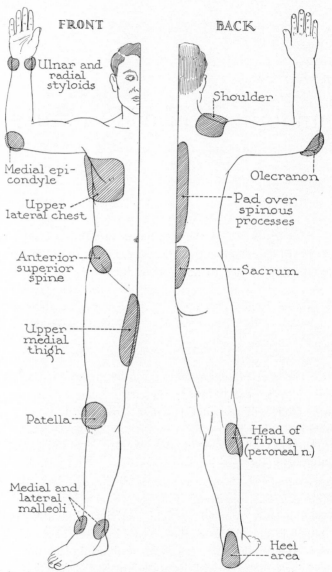

FRONT   BACK

Ulnar and radial styloids

Shoulder

Medial epicondyle

Olecranon

Upper lateral chest

Pad over spinous processes

Anterior superior spine

Sacrum

Upper medial thigh

Patella

Head of fibula (peroneal n.)

Medial and lateral malleoli

Heel area

FIG. 7.—Areas which should be carefully protected by felt, rubber or cotton pads before incorporating them in a plaster cast.

40

more ready to resume their regular work and take over the family and community responsibilities which the injury temporarily interrupted.

With rare exceptions, yucca board or single splints (aluminum, wire, basket) of any kind should be used only in first aid or emergency procedures. This applies in war as well as in civilian practice. Yucca board splints are most unsatisfactory in the treatment of fractures of the long bones. They do not fit the contour of the limb accurately and can be applied only to one

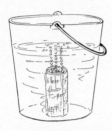 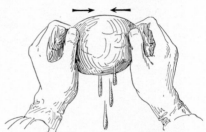

Roll of plaster placed on end in pail of water. Roll saturated when bubbles cease to appear.

Excess water squeezed from plaster roll by pushing both ends towards the middle. Do not twist.

FIG. 8.—Correct handling of the plaster roll.

side of the limb. Motion between the fracture fragments, with displacement, occurs all too often.

For the average fracture, closely fitted plaster casts, accurately molded to the contour of the limb, with padding over the bony prominences, are by far the safest and most adequate for maintaining immobilization (Fig. 7). These plaster casts may be applied as anterior and posterior molded splints or as circular plaster dressings (Figs. 8 and 9). Molded plaster splints without circular plaster bandages have two distinct advantages: (1) the dressings may be easily loosened by cutting the gauze bandage, if the swelling becomes sufficiently great to endanger circulation in the extremity, and (2) they may be readily tightened by application of additional bandage as the swelling subsides.

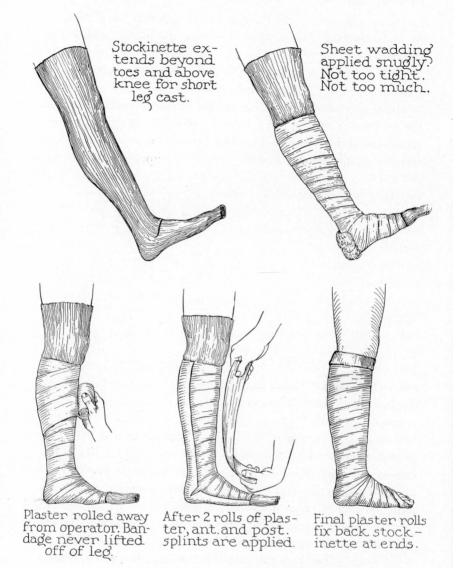

Stockinette extends beyond toes and above knee for short leg cast.

Sheet wadding applied snugly. Not too tight. Not too much.

Plaster rolled away from operator. Bandage never lifted off of leg.

After 2 rolls of plaster, ant. and post. splints are applied.

Final plaster rolls fix back stockinette at ends.

FIG. 9.—Technique of application of plaster cast.

The authors rarely use circular plaster casts applied directly to the skin. The use of felt and sheet wadding for padding is dependent upon the amount of swelling expected; in the absence of swelling the plaster may be applied snugly over stockinette, with minimal padding for bony prominences.

Metal pins placed above and below the fracture site, but not sufficiently close to the fracture to enter the hematoma, may be incorporated in circular plaster dressings and thus provide complete immobilization without the necessity of stopping motion in the adjacent joints. However, if no skeletal fixation is used (by means of pins or Kirschner or threaded wires), the plaster cast should extend well beyond the adjacent articulation, both above and below the site of fracture, in order to assure adequate immobilization (Fig. 10).

The treatment of fractures, with the patient at bed rest, by continuous traction on metal frames or with the aid of the Thomas splint (with a Pierson attachment to permit knee joint motion) has proved to be highly efficient in maintaining reduction and in obtaining a good functional end-result. The disadvantages of continuous traction over a period of four to 12 weeks have already been mentioned. Keeping a patient flat on his back for many weeks is to be deplored, unless other equally efficient, but less confining, methods of immobilization are not possible.

INTERNAL FIXATION OF FRACTURES may be used if there are suitable indications. Open reduction of fractures should not be carried out when it is possible to obtain and maintain a satisfactory re-position of the fragments by some closed method. The principal objections to open reduction are:

1. Danger of contamination, with resultant infection at the site of the fracture.
2. Interference with the first stage of fracture healing, caused by loss of the hematoma through the wound.

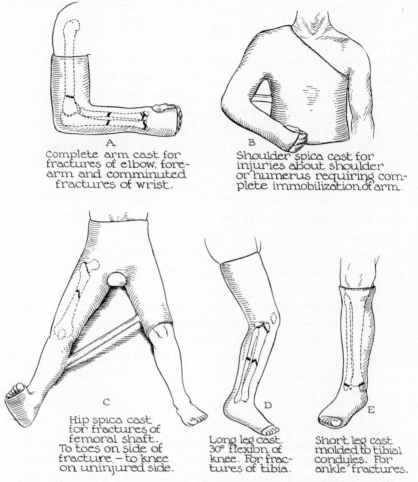

A.
Complete arm cast for fractures of elbow, forearm and comminuted fractures of wrist.

B.
Shoulder spica cast for injuries about shoulder or humerus requiring complete immobilization of arm.

C.
Hip spica cast for fractures of femoral shaft. To toes on side of fracture — to knee on uninjured side.

D.
Long leg cast. 30° flexion of knee. For fractures of tibia.

E.
Short leg cast molded to tibial condyles. For ankle fractures.

FIG. 10.—Several types of plaster cast and some of the fractures for which they may be indicated. Apply cast with the knee in slight flexion. The problem of restoring motion in stiff knees will be greatly lessened if this recommendation is followed.

44

3. Stripping of periosteum, which may devitalize the ends of the fracture fragments and cause delayed union or non-union.

Foreign body reactions in the tissues are minimal when vitallium or stainless steel is used for internal fixation. When metal fixation is necessary these substances are well tolerated by bones. They are available in the form of pins, screws and plates. Internal fixation should be reserved for those fractures in which there is: (1) evidence of injury to major nerves or blood vessels, requiring surgical repair of these structures; (2) interposition of muscle or other soft tissue structures between the fragments, so that closed reduction could not be obtained; (3) open fracture; (4) after osteotomy for the correction of a united fracture in malposition; (5) unstable oblique fracture, or (6) need to avoid prolonged recumbency.

The following means of obtaining internal fixation have been used:

1. Smith-Petersen or Cubbins-Callahan-Scuderi nails, for intracapsular hip fractures.
2. Multiple wires drilled directly through the skin and across the fracture line, penetrating both fracture fragments after reduction has been obtained. Recommended only if wires are cut off beneath the skin.
3. Long screws crossing the fracture line and binding the fragments together.
4. Metal plates of vitallium or stainless steel fitted accurately across the fracture line after reduction and attached by screws which pass through the one cortex and engage the opposite cortex of the bone. The slotted plate is recommended because it permits the maintenance of contact between the fragments in spite of absorption at the bone ends.
5. A special metal plate used in the treatment of intertrochanteric fractures and consisting of a flange portion

that enters the neck of the femur while the plate is attached by screws to the subtrochanteric shaft.

6. Metal bands, which too often are either too loose to maintain good immobilization of the fragments or so tight that
they constrict and produce pressure necrosis, are recom-

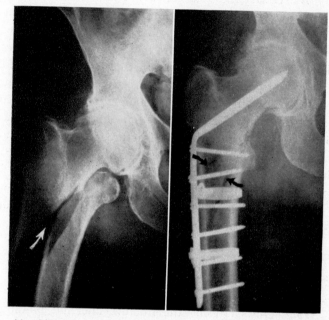

FIG. 11.—Oblique fracture of the femur through the level of the lesser
trochanter. This fracture may be adequately immobilized with use of a blade
plate as illustrated. A Parham band may be used in addition to approximate
the fragments more securely, particularly for atrophic or pathologic bone.

mended only for certain complicated fractures (Fig. 11).

7. Intramedullary rods of the solid diamond, cloverleaf or
round type have a wide application, particularly for fractures of the femur.

Each individual case must be treated on its own merits. If an
unstable fracture has been opened and it is necessary to expose

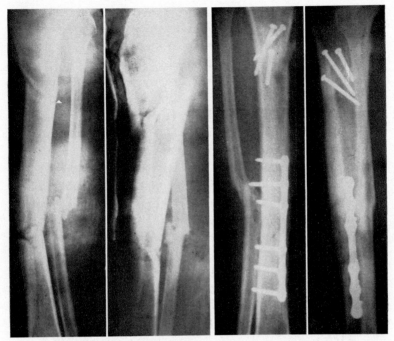

F‍IG. 12 *(left)*.—Double fractures of the tibia with posterior displacement at the proximal and medial angulation at the distal fracture site. Skeletal traction through the lower end of the tibia will distract the distal fragments and not influence the upper fracture.

F‍IG. 13 *(right)*.—Same case as preceding. Normal re-position of fragments obtained by use of multiple screws above and a metal plate below. Excellent functional result was obtained.

47

the fracture ends in order to assure a thorough débridement, an experienced surgeon will be entirely justified in inserting a plate, screws, threaded wires, or an intramedullary rod (Fig. 41), to maintain the position (Figs. 12 and 13). The wound should then be sutured loosely without drainage, thus converting it into a closed fracture whenever this is possible.

Maintenance of reduction by internal fixation is in some few cases the only satisfactory means which will afford a reasonable chance of union and at the same time permit functional activity. Intracapsular fracture of the neck of the femur is the best example. After reduction, this fracture may be adequately immobilized by means of the Smith-Petersen three-flange, or the Cubbins-Callahan-Scuderi two-flange, nail or by means of screws or threaded pins. During World War II we were not able to obtain threaded wires which could be relied upon. Some were brittle and fragmented in the tissues. Others were soft and would bend like stovepipe wire. We are now using the Smith-Petersen nail and consider it the most consistently satisfactory method of internal fixation of intracapsular fractures of the hip.

CHAPTER VIII

General Principles of Care

Nurses who have had good orthopedic experience are essential for thoroughly satisfactory care of patients presenting major fracture problems. However, if the surgeon is alert to all the possibilities of complications that may occur in these cases, he will not depend entirely on the nurses but will supervise their work and make certain that fundamental principles are actually put into practice in the daily care of his patients. Unless given the benefit of excellent nursing care, most elderly patients and many younger ones who are so badly injured or so completely immobilized that they are unable to shift from one position to another will develop trophic or pressure ulcers over such bony prominences as the sacrum or greater trochanter. Except when there are definite contraindications, all patients must be turned to the prone position for at least one hour twice each day if they are not able freely to change position for themselves. If the fracture is of the hip, femur or spine, the patient should be turned with the greatest of skill to avoid inflicting unnecessary pain, breaking the cast or displacing fracture fragments. A competent orderly or nurse will learn the technique quickly. Patients are turned most easily by means of a draw sheet. Upon the draw sheet they can be gently dragged to one side of the bed. When the edges of the draw sheet are then grasped firmly and lifted evenly, the patient will be rolled without torsion of spine or hips. If the cast extends down on the legs, a second attendant must *lift* the cast leg, to protect the opposite leg or hip from undue stress and weight and also to prevent the cast from breaking at the groin. When the patient is in certain positions, the edges of a large cast will produce pressure on soft parts. This pressure can be minimized or entirely relieved by intelligent arrangement of pillows under the extremity or under the trunk.

In the extremity that is being subjected to traction or is encased in plaster casts, circulation may become impaired through pressure from the splint or the traction apparatus or from the swelling of the contused tissues. No extremity should be so completely covered with plaster or with any other immobilizing apparatus that the fingers and toes are not exposed so that they may be frequently observed. Moderate swelling can usually be controlled by adequate splitting along one margin of the cast, and elevation of the extremity. Cyanosis, pain and disturbed sensation in the digits will be produced by any serious complication within the cast which threatens to interfere with the circulation of the extremity. Severe and intractable pain in an extremity which is encased in a plaster cast, or in any type of splint, should not be ignored. If the pain is not relieved by adjustment of the cast or splint, it is most unwise to attempt to eliminate this warning signal by means of morphine until one has ascertained beyond any doubt that pressure within the cast against a nerve, blood vessel or bony prominence is not the cause of the patient's suffering. When there is any reasonable doubt, the cast should be sacrificed, if necessary, in order to inspect the entire extremity. When a cast is split to relieve a circulatory disturbance, the wise surgeon will make certain that all strands of the crinoline or of bandages beneath the plaster have been cut through. A few remaining strands of crinoline or sheet

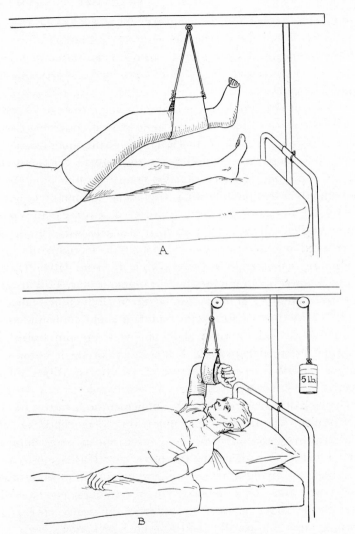

A

B

FIG. 14.—Excessive swelling of an extremity immobilized in a plaster dressing may be minimized by adequate suspension of the part.

wadding may cause sufficient constriction to lead to necrosis or
at least to Volkmann's ischemic paralysis. Elevation of an extremity by means of suspension to an overhead frame may control or prevent marked edema (Fig. 14). This is superior to elevation on pillows.

As a result either of direct pressure on nerve roots or of reflex
action, fractures of the pelvis or spine may produce *ileus* with
marked *abdominal distention*. Distention of the small bowel not
only produces severe discomfort for the patient but may em-
barrass respiration and, occasionally, contribute to a fatal result.
Abdominal distention following any major trauma requires a
differential diagnosis between rupture of a viscus and post-
traumatic ileus. Ileus, in the absence of a ruptured viscus, can
be relieved in most instances by means of a rectal tube and
stimulating enemas. In resistant cases the stimulating enema
can be followed in 15 minutes by $\frac{1}{2}$ ampule of 1:2,000 Pitressin.
The remaining $\frac{1}{2}$ ampule can be given 30 minutes later, if
needed. Heat, in the form either of hot, moist fomentation or
of an electric pad over the abdomen, will sometimes assist in
restoring intestinal peristalsis. Acute gastric or small bowel distention may be relieved by the use of a Levin or Miller-Abbott
tube.

The lack of activity caused by confinement in a cast or in bed
may result in constipation, and unless this is controlled by suitable measures, *fecal impaction* may occur and be most unpleas-
ant for both the patient and the physician. This is most easily
prevented by giving 1 oz. of mineral oil morning or evening
until bowel function is regular. An oil retention enema given
every second day, followed by a warm tap water enema the
morning after, will usually control severe obstipation.

CHAPTER IX

Rate of Healing of Fractures

MANY factors affect the rate of healing of fractures. Cellular activity, and hence tissue repair, is more rapid in young children than in elderly individuals.

The type of fracture also determines to some extent the rate of healing. Long oblique or comminuted fractures which have extensive fracture surfaces will heal more slowly than accurately reduced transverse fractures of the same bone.

Disturbed blood supply to one or more fragments is second only to poor reduction and inadequate or insufficiently prolonged immobilization as a cause of delayed union or nonunion. This is most often observed in fractures of the neck of the femur, navicular bone and talus, fractures of joint surfaces with detachment of fragments causing inadequate vascular supply and comminuted fractures in which segments may be completely stripped of periosteum. Infection at the fracture site may lead to sequestration of the ends of the fragments, causing marked delay and, not infrequently, nonunion. In general, fractures of small bones unite more rapidly than do those of larger bones.

Fractures of flat bones such as the pelvis, the ribs and the scapula heal rapidly, and nonunion is exceedingly rare. In the

TABLE 2.—APPROXIMATE IMMOBILIZATION NECESSARY FOR UNION

FRACTURE SITE	No. OF WEEKS	
	Children	Adults
Phalanx	3	3
Metacarpal	6	6
Carpal	Rare	6
Scaphoid	Rare	10, or until x-ray shows union
Radius and ulna	6–8	10–12
Humerus		
supracondylar	6	8
midshaft	6	8–12
proximal—impacted	3	3 (early motion)
—displaced	6	6–8
Clavicle	4	6
Vertebra	16	16
Pelvis	4	6
Femur		
intracapsular	16	24
intertrochanteric	6	10–12
shaft	8–10	18
supracondylar	6–8	12–15
Tibia		
proximal	6	8–10
shaft	8–10	14–20
malleolus	6	6
Calcaneus	10	12–16
Metatarsal	6	6
Toes	3	3

ribs this is true in spite of the impossibility of obtaining complete immobilization because of movement in respiration.

Fractures that occur toward the ends of the long bones, where the cortex is less thick and the cancellous bone is more abundant, heal more rapidly than do fractures of the mid-shaft, where the bone is less vascular and cancellous.

CHAPTER X

After-Treatment of Fractures

WHEN functional activity has been maintained to the fullest possible extent during the period of immobilization of the fracture fragments, management after the fracture heals is relatively simple. The functional activity should include constant exercise of all joints where motion can be permitted during the period of immobilization without jeopardizing the patient's chances of obtaining union of the fracture. Thus it is possible to secure adequate immobilization of Colles' type fracture while still permitting and encouraging free motion of all of the fingers, the thumb and the shoulder. Active, vigorous motion should not only be permitted but be insisted on. A few feeble or perfunctory movements of the fingers each day is the average patient's concept of exercising the hand. Firm grasping and opening and closing the hand will cause some pain, and few patients will follow instructions unless they are repeated often and adequately explained or demonstrated. Each patient must be made to understand why it is so important to use all the strength possible for each individual finger motion. In injury to a lower extremity requiring cast immobilization, quadriceps and gluteus medius exercises should be carried out at regular intervals each day

(Fig. 15). This will minimize atrophy of disuse and thereby shorten the period of convalescence.

After the cast has been removed and union has been definitely established, physical therapy may aid in further restoration of complete physiologic function. The *physical therapy should not*

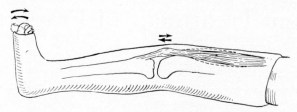

A. Quadriceps exercises in long leg cast.
Toe exercises by flexion and extension.

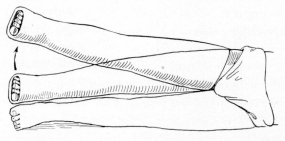

B.   Gluteus medius exercises in long leg cast

FIG. 15.—Atrophy of the quadriceps muscle should be combated by active contractions of the muscle during the period of immobilization. Maintenance of gluteus medius muscle power facilitates early return of normal walking following healing of fractures in the lower extremity.

include passive stretching of finger joints which have become partially stiffened due to immobilization. Such forced stretching not only produces pain, with an accompanying anxiety state, but may lead to more prolonged hyperemia and fibrosis, with further limitation of joint motion. Occasionally, also, it will be followed by the development of calcification or ossification around or within the capsule of the joint. This is seen most often at the elbow, but can occur in the shoulder, knee, ankle or the hip joint.

The primary aim of physical therapy should be to assist in the restoration of good circulatory exchange. The swelling which follows long immobilization of an extremity can be prevented or minimized by the use of a compression elastic bandage or an Unna paste boot. Functional activity, however, will do more to restore the circulation than will any mechanical or passive procedure. Radiant heat, the whirlpool bath, contrast bath and diathermy may be useful in certain cases. Each of these procedures, with the possible exception of the whirlpool bath, which in itself provides the principle not only of heat but of massage (owing to the motion of the water), should be followed by intelligent massage. Intelligent massage never produces pain; it is soothing and should be directed toward the heart from the most distal portion of an extremity. Heat in any form produces capillary and arterial dilatation. This, in effect, increases the hyperemia temporarily. Massage overcomes the local congestion, empties the superficial capillaries and helps to produce a directional flow of lymph. With rare exceptions, therefore, massage should accompany or follow the application of direct heat to an extremity or to any part of the body surface.

Active motion is most important in the after-care of a fracture. It should be carried out by the patient under the supervision and, if necessary, at the insistence of the physical therapist. Active motion will restore power to the muscles, freedom to the adherent tendons and mobility to the joints which may have become partially stiffened because of the long immobilization. Active motion will not tear the joint capsule or injure other tissues, whereas passive stretching is attended by this danger.

Resistive active exercise, repeated at regular intervals against progressively increasing resistance, is the most effective form of treatment for restoration of muscle strength and joint mobility. The method is of particular value for disuse atrophy of the quadriceps mechanism (Fig. 16). The exercise consists of 75 repetitions at one exercise period daily. These are divided into five series of 15 repetitions each with a short rest period between each series. The poundage is determined weekly. At first the load consists of the amount of weight with which the patient can just

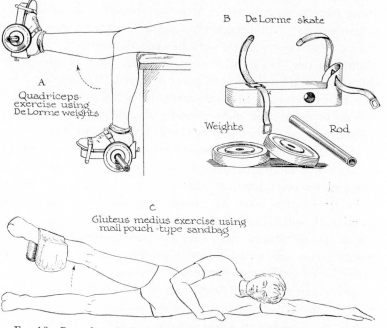

FIG. 16.—Proved method of restoring both volume and power to atrophied muscles by a program of weight-lifting as described by DeLorme.

extend the knee. At the end of the last treatment period of the first week, additional weights are added gradually to determine the load which will still permit full active extension of the knee. This poundage will then be the load for the second week. The load is increased each week, requiring a constantly greater effort on the part of the quadriceps muscle. Remarkable results have been obtained with this method in patients with severe simple atrophy and also in those with partially unstable joints. The principle is applicable to any muscle group.

Manipulation under an anesthetic is at times necessary in order to break up actual fibrous bands which may freeze the quadriceps tendon or may produce adhesions within the quadriceps bursa or around the shoulder—adhesions which may be too strong for the patient to overcome by means of active motion and use of the extremity. Following any manipulation, every effort should be made to encourage the patient to use the extremity actively. It should be moved through as wide a range of joint motion as possible, many times each day. A roentgenogram should be taken after each manipulation to ascertain whether a fracture or dislocation has occurred.

Manipulation of the elbow is contraindicated. Experience has proved that forceful stretching of this joint usually results in further ankylosis and disability.

Application of a brace for the spine or for a lower extremity is often advisable following the healing of a fracture. A well fitted brace will often permit early weight-bearing, and it will protect the recently healed fracture against re-fracture or angulation. Braces are of value psychologically when they afford a sense of security, and the patient is thus enabled to use an extremity which otherwise might become even more atrophic.

CHAPTER XI

Open and Infected Fractures

A N OPEN fracture constitutes one of the most serious of all emergencies. The involved bone is exposed through the skin and must be considered to be potentially infected. The need for prompt and adequate surgical care is as urgent as that for the treatment of acute appendicitis, a ruptured spleen or perforation of a peptic ulcer. Delay in treatment of an open fracture may result in infection, with osteomyelitis, septicemia, nonunion, prolonged invalidism, loss of a limb or death (Fig. 17). Two primary considerations must be kept in mind in planning the management of open fractures. The first is prevention or treatment of shock, for the immediate preservation of life. Second is the prevention of infection in the wound (Fig. 18).

The recommended treatment of open fractures is outlined.

EMERGENCY CARE AT SITE OF ACCIDENT

1. Give morphine sulfate, gr. ¼, for pain *unless there is a head injury*. Omit morphine if the patient is a small child.
2. Treat shock—control bleeding by pressure dressing and protect patient from heat loss.
3. Clamp the severed superficial blood vessels that are not controlled by a pressure dressing.

4. Apply an adequate splint *before moving the patient*. This will lessen shock and prevent further damage to soft tissues.

5. Transport the patient to a hospital without unnecessary

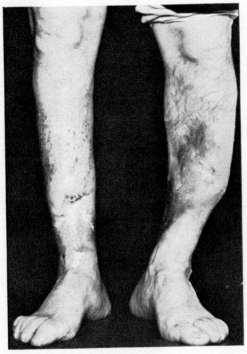

Fig. 17.—Fractures of both tibiae with persistent infection, drainage and nonunion seven years after injury.

delay—on a stretcher if the spine, pelvis, femur or tibia is involved or if the patient is unconscious.

6. Apply tourniquets only when absolutely necessary to stop hemorrhage. They are dangerous, and may be overlooked, resulting in gangrene.

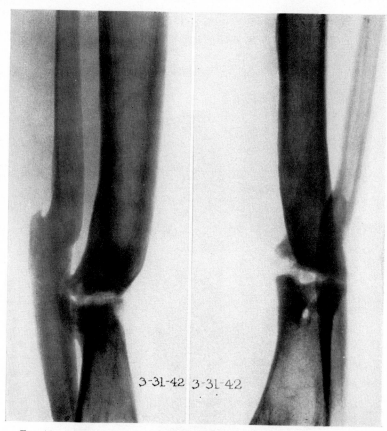

3-31-42 3-31-42

Fig. 18.—Infected open fracture of the tibia, ununited after seven years.

HOSPITAL CARE

1. Continue treatment of shock while the operating room is being prepared. Apply warm blankets and hot water bottles. Administer adequate amounts of plasma, whole blood or glucose and saline.

   In deep shock, give continuous blood plasma or whole blood, or both. Do not stop after one transfusion if shock is not relieved. Give oxygen by nasal catheter.

   Search for evidence of other injuries—to the brain, a ruptured viscus or internal hemorrhage.

2. Give penicillin, 600,000 units intramuscularly, and daily thereafter until the temperature has been normal for 48 hours.

3. As soon as the patient's condition permits, excise the wound in the operating room (Fig. 19).

   a) Place the leg on a fracture table in the traction stirrups, but without traction.

   b) Continue the administration of fluids intravenously if they are needed.

   c) Obtain roentgenograms while the operator scrubs his hands for 10 minutes and dons sterile gown and gloves. The nose and mouth must be covered.

   d) Apply skeletal traction, if indicated.

   e) Scrub the skin for 10 minutes with white soap and sterile cotton while protecting the open wound with a sterile towel.

   f) The operator should change his gloves. Block off the prepared area with sterile towels and wash the interior of the wound for 10 minutes, or longer, using white soap or a detergent and water. Irrigate from below upward with large volumes of warm, sterile saline. Again change gloves; then drape the wound.

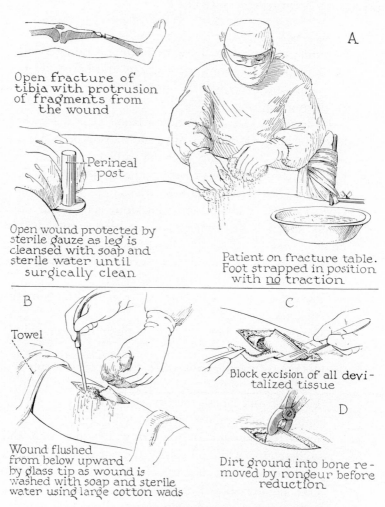

Open fracture of tibia with protrusion of fragments from the wound

Perineal post

Open wound protected by sterile gauze as leg is cleansed with soap and sterile water until surgically clean

A

Patient on fracture table. Foot strapped in position with <u>no</u> traction

B

Towel

Wound flushed from below upward by glass tip as wound is washed with soap and sterile water using large cotton wads

C

Block excision of all devitalized tissue

D

Dirt ground into bone removed by rongeur before reduction

FIG. 19.—Care of the open fracture.

g) Excise the walls of the wound. Start from the skin and go down (débridement). Obtain hemostasis.

h) Rongeur away all grossly contaminated bone.

i) Remove only the small detached fragments, *no* large fragments.

j) Reduce the fracture, and consider internal fixation if the fragments are unstable. Fixation may be obtained by skeletal pins placed well above and below the fracture, with incorporation in plaster.

k) Repair severed tendons and nerves. If infection appears probable, a minimal number of interrupted sutures should be used for approximation.

4. Shall the wound be sutured or packed open?

a) Close the wound without tension if patient is treated within six to eight hours after injury.

Bury little plain catgut. Do not bury chromic sutures. Do not suture muscles or fascia.

Make parallel skin incisions to effect closure if necessary.

Apply split skin grafts to the secondary wounds.

b) Spread the wound open with petrolatum-impregnated gauze *if* the patient is seen after eight hours or if it is the surgeon's opinion that the wound should not be closed, even though less than eight hours have elapsed before excision. (Do not *pack* wound.) The open method should be compulsory if (1) the surgeon is not experienced in open fracture surgery or (2) the patient must be immediately evacuated after primary treatment.

5 Immobilize the fracture adequately with plaster dressing (Fig. 20) and permit the patient to be ambulatory on crutches, if at all possible. The multiple pin method, in conjunction with plaster or external metal bar, leaving all

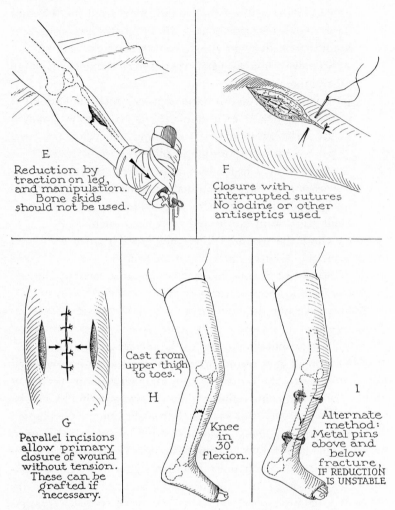

E

Reduction by traction on leg, and manipulation. Bone skids should not be used.

F

Closure with interrupted sutures No iodine or other antiseptics used

G

Parallel incisions allow primary closure of wound without tension. These can be grafted if necessary.

H

Cast from upper thigh to toes.

Knee in 30° flexion.

I

Alternate method: Metal pins above and below fracture, IF REDUCTION IS UNSTABLE

FIG. 20.—Primary closure after cleansing, débriding and reducing an open fracture of the tibia.

joints free, may be used by those experienced in the technique. Unstable open fractures that cannot be adequately immobilized by plaster casts alone may be splinted internally with nonirritating metal plates and screws, or an intramedullary rod.

6. Give tetanus antitoxin, 3,000 international units, or a 0.5 cc. booster dose of tetanus toxoid if the patient has previously been immunized.

7. If the wound is contaminated with dirt from the highway or cultivated fields, give gas bacillus antitoxin.

8. Penicillin therapy, as recommended, may be supplemented by the oral administration of aureomycin, terramycin or chloramphenicol.

Too much emphasis cannot be placed on the importance of performing an adequate débridement. This does not mean the mere cutting away of skin margins, as so many students are led to believe from inadequate descriptions of this procedure in their textbooks. It means the excision of all devitalized and contaminated tissues except major nerves and blood vessels. The use in the wound of iodine, benzine or other strong antiseptics which devitalize living cells and predispose them to infection is definitely condemned. The use of the sulfonamides, penicillin or other chemotherapeutic agents cannot compensate for inadequate excision of the wound. It has been shown by comparable series of cases that unless adequate débridement is performed, the incidence of infection in open wounds treated within eight hours is not much lowered by local use of sulfonamides or any antibiotic.

On few medical questions have there been so many sharply divided opinions as are held today regarding the treatment of open fractures. The discussions center around two acceptable plans of management, already outlined: (1) primary closure of the wound, and (2) the open method. It is to be noted that either of these methods must be preceded by a thorough cleansing and adequate débridement and that either should be attended by accurate reduction of the fracture and the best possible fixation of the reduced fragments while preserving, whenever possible, ambulation of the patient.

In civilian practice, experience has shown that primary closure may be routinely performed with excellent results when the patient appears for treatment within six to eight hours after injury and that the open method is preferable when more than eight hours have elapsed. The open method is safer and has been universally adopted under war conditions, where *more than 50 per cent of all major casualties* include at least one open fracture. Too often the war wound will have been invaded by organisms before initial treatment is possible, and the soldier must be evacuated to the rear immediately after primary treatment of the area of the compound trauma. The reports of Trueta, who used the Orr petrolatum pack method in all compound wounds and fractures occurring in the Republican armies during the war in Spain, are indeed enlightening. Good results were obtained in 976 of 1,073 cases.

For the physician who has had little actual experience and training in fracture management and cannot perform a skilful cleansing and débridement of the wound or is not able to provide adequate after-care of the patient, the open method is undoubtedly safer under all circumstances.

Primary closure of open fractures has certain advantages:

1. This method, when successful, turns open into closed fractures.

2. Both primary and secondary infection is avoided, and osteomyelitis is prevented.

3. Healing of soft tissues is complete in 10 to 12 days.

4. The scar is linear and relatively nonadherent.

5. The hospitalization period is shortened.

6. The total period of disability is lessened.

Contraindications to primary closure of open fracture wounds may be summarized as follows:

1. Wounds over eight to 10 hours old.
2. Wounds widely contused.
3. Prevalence of gas organisms in the geographic area, with definite contamination of the wound.
4. Inadequate débridement owing to presence in the wound of major vessels and nerves.
5. Tissues under tension. (These may be relaxed by incision of the skin at a distance from the wound.)
6. All war wounds, which are often multiple, including open fractures.

Early secondary closure, carried out five to 10 days after the original débridement, is a valuable recent development in the treatment of open fractures. It is indicated when the wound is granulating with minimal suppuration and without deep sinus formation.

Patients with open fractures who arrive at the hospital for care after suppuration is definitely established, or too long after injury to permit primary closure, should be treated by the open method.

OPEN METHOD OF TREATMENT OF INFECTED
OPEN FRACTURES

1. Use regional or general anesthesia.
2. Place the patient on the fracture table, in traction, if necessary.
3. Establish adequate drainage of pus, opening all recesses.
4. Remove small sequestra and foreign bodies.
5. Insert petrolatum-impregnated gauze into all recesses of the wound.
6. Apply a plaster of paris cast, including the joints above and below. The multiple pin method may be used to

avoid immobilization of already stiff joints and to permit early ambulation or evacuation.

7. Give tetanus and gas antitoxin, unless previously administered.

8. Penicillin, 600,000 units daily, should be started. In severe infection, other antibiotics should also be given in adequate doses.

9. Do not disturb the cast for six weeks unless there is evidence of complication, such as tetanus or gas infection. Odor beneath the plaster is not an indication for frequent changing of cast.

10. Technique of changing cast and wound dressing:

   a) Use general or regional anesthesia.

   b) Remove the cast and petrolatum gauze pack.

   c) Use sterile precautions—mask, gown, gloves.

   d) Free wound of pus. Remove additional sequestra.

   e) Consider secondary closure of wound by suture or split thickness skin graft. This is indicated if the wound is granulating cleanly.

Patients treated by the open method are comfortable, cheerful and eat well. If they become restless, refuse food and *the pulse becomes rapid* or the temperature elevated, the presence of gas or tetanus infection must be suspected.

GAS GANGRENE.—The bacteria which cause gas gangrene do not multiply or become clinically virulent in the presence of an abundant supply of oxygen. They multiply and overpower the resistance of living tissue only when they are entrenched in dirt that is deep in a wound or embedded in devitalized tissue which is deprived of most or all of its blood supply. Early cleansing and excision of a contaminated wound will, in almost all cases, prevent infection by these anaerobic organisms. They cannot thrive in a clean wound in the presence of a rich blood supply. Complete débridement of all contaminated wounds as early as possible is of greater importance than the injection of any amount of the usual antitoxin prepared from gas-forming bacteria. Use of antitoxin is an approved prophylactic measure in the treatment of open fractures, especially when such injuries occur in regions known to harbor these organisms in the soil. The physician, however, must not be lulled into a feeling of false security, regardless of how much antibiotic or antitoxin he has used. They do not take the place of skilful and adequate surgery.

The diagnosis of gas gangrene is indicated by:

1. A rising pulse rate.
2. Fever.
3. Marked apprehension.
4. Pain, swelling and crepitation in the soft tissues.
5. A thin, watery exudate.
6. Exceedingly foul odor of the wound.

TREATMENT OF GAS GANGRENE

1. Operate immediately to establish free drainage by means of multiple and adequate incisions through the skin and fascia, made in the long axis of the limb.
2. Remove any sutures previously inserted in the wound.
3. Excise all definitely gangrenous muscle and fascia.
4. Irrigate continuously for 12 hours with a solution of equal parts of potassium permanganate (1:10,000 dilution) and hydrogen peroxide. Repeat intermittently until the infection is controlled.
5. Give full doses of sulfonamide and aureomycin by mouth and penicillin by intramuscular injection.
6. Give 60,000 units of antitoxin intravenously and continue with 30,000 units daily while the toxemia persists.
7. Roentgen therapy should be tried. The dosage should be 75–100 roentgen units, given through each of two or more portals daily for three days.
8. Do not amputate unless massive gangrene develops. If

amputation becomes necessary, apply a tourniquet, amputate and leave the wound unsutured. Apply traction to skin within a few days.

TETANUS.—Tetanus infection can be prevented, in almost all cases, either by good surgery or by a combination of surgery and antitoxin. Three thousand international units of antitoxin or 0.5 cc. of toxoid should be given as soon as possible after the wound is inflicted. Before receiving the antitoxin, each subject must be tested for sensitivity to horse serum and, if necessary, desensitized.

The symptoms of tetanus usually begin with twitching in the region of the wound, followed by muscular rigidity in the extremity and later throughout the body. Early occurrence of reflex spasms and severe convulsions make the prognosis exceedingly poor.

TREATMENT OF TETANUS INFECTION

1. Tetanus antitoxin, 200,000 international units, should be injected intravenously.
2. If the patient survives, 50,000 units should be given every seven days until all reflex spasms subside.
3. The spasms may be controlled by Avertin or paraldehyde.
4. If the local wound is small, it should be excised one hour after the surrounding tissues have been infiltrated with tetanus antitoxin.
5. Penicillin, 600,000 units twice daily, should be given.

SUMMARY

The well trained surgeon in civilian practice can and should cleanse, débride and close all wounds of open fractures seen within eight hours of injury. War wounds may have to be treated by physicians who have not had wide training in surgical technique and the principles of thorough cleansing and débridement of contaminated wounds or the discipline needed in the management of major fractures. Under these circumstances, the wounds should be washed, cleansed with warm normal saline solution, débrided as well as possible, spread open with petrolatum-impregnated gauze and immobilized. The patient should be transported as soon as possible to a medical center for further treatment of the fracture. Penicillin should be given in doses of 600,000 units daily and other antibiotics as indicated.

Each doubtful case, with proper primary treatment by the open method, should be observed closely during the first two weeks to determine whether early secondary closure is justified.

It would be well for all of us to remember that during the past two decades tremendous progress has been made in methods of treatment of fractures. Some of the principles of both open and closed fracture surgery that were acceptable in 1918 are as out of date today as are the weapons of war that were used by our first A.E.F. in France. We should be prepared to give our patients the highest type of medical and surgical care. When the services of more experienced colleagues are available, they should be solicited to provide the best treatment for difficult or open fractures.

CHAPTER XII

Delayed Union and Nonunion

SOME of the reasons for delayed union or nonunion of fractures have been discussed in Chapters VII and IX. These consist of (1) inaccurate reduction, (2) inadequate immobilization, (3) failure to maintain immobilization for a sufficient length of time, and (4) distraction with the fragments held apart. Disturbance of the blood supply locally, through the tearing of nutrient arteries, is the fifth common cause of delayed union or nonunion.

Glandular or mineral metabolic deficiencies are seldom responsible for failures of union, and when such failures occur, the surgeon will do well to examine critically his own method of dealing with the local fracture. Vitamin substances, calcium, parathormone and other mineral or endocrine products *are of no value* in the treatment of fractures, except in the rare instances in which there is definitely a deficiency, as in rickets or osteomalacia. In the clinically normal and healthy individual there is no indication whatever for administering these substances in massive doses. They may, in fact, be contraindicated. Both calcium and vitamin D have been shown experimentally to be harmful when given in amounts greater than needed to maintain optimal nutrition.

Directives in the treatment of delayed union may be listed as follows:

1. Prolong the period of immobilization.

2. Ascertain that reduction and immobilization are adequate.

3. Permit the bone to perform work, such as weight-bearing, using a walking iron in the cast.

4. Remove sequestra and attempt both surgically and by chemotherapy to heal infection, if present.

5. Unless there is definite constitutional evidence of a deficiency, do not give large doses of vitamin D, calcium, parathormone or other mineral and endocrine products.

The difference between nonunion and delayed union is not always clearly demonstrable. If union fails to take place after a prolonged period of adequate immobilization and there are no other discernible factors which can be corrected in order to bring about union spontaneously, the diagnosis of nonunion is justified. When there is nonunion, either because of poor management of the fracture from the beginning or because of factors which were beyond control of the surgeon, the stimulus to repair at the site of the fracture will have been dissipated. Some physicians attempt to obtain union in these cases by performing an open operation and fixing the fragments together with wire or applying a metal plate. Although this method is occasionally successful, a higher percentage of unions will result if autogenous bone is placed as an inlay or onlay graft across the fracture site. The autogenous bone may be expected to become attached to and unite the fracture fragments. A metal plate or an intramedullary rod (Fig. 21) in combination with a bone graft may assure the maintenance of reduction in unstable fractures or in fractures that tend to angulation after the application of the plaster cast, as those of the femur, humerus, radius and ulna. The onlay graft may be secured in position by suturing the surrounding soft tissues, or by means of metal screws, and if the bone graft is large and strong this serves the dual purpose of stimulating osteogenesis and holding the fragments firmly together (Fig. 22).

The intermediary fibrous callus helps to maintain alignment of the fragments and should not be excised unless it is necessary

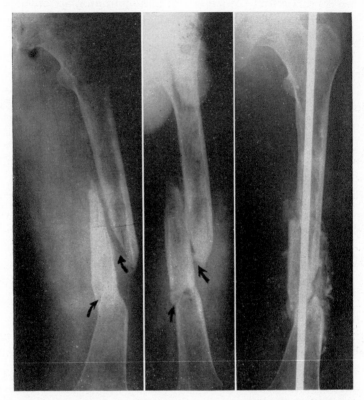

Fig. 21.—Nonunion of both sites of a segmental fracture of the middle third of the femur treated with an intramedullary rod and both cortical and cancellous bone grafts taken from the patient's ilium. This is another definite indication for use of the intramedullary rod.

to break up such fibrous union in order to obtain more accurate apposition and alignment of the fragments. This fibrous callus constitutes one stage of union and, if the bone grafts become attached, will usually proceed to complete ossification.

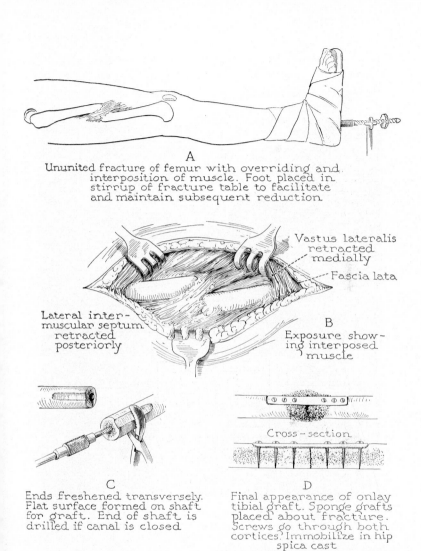

A

Ununited fracture of femur with overriding and interposition of muscle. Foot placed in stirrup of fracture table to facilitate and maintain subsequent reduction

Vastus lateralis retracted medially

Fascia lata

Lateral inter- muscular septum retracted posteriorly

B

Exposure show- ing interposed muscle

Cross-section

C

Ends freshened transversely. Flat surface formed on shaft for graft. End of shaft is drilled if canal is closed

D

Final appearance of onlay tibial graft. Sponge grafts placed about fracture. Screws go through both cortices. Immobilize in hip spica cast

FIG. 22.—Treatment of nonunion and malposition of fracture of the femur. The same procedure may be used to obtain fixation and osteosynthesis after correction of malunion.

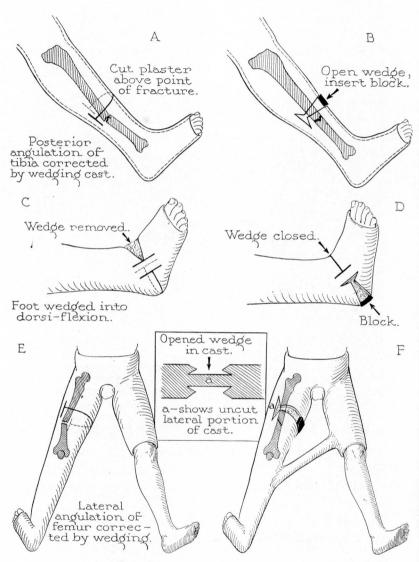

A

Cut plaster
above point
of fracture.

Posterior
angulation of
tibia corrected
by wedging cast.

B

Open wedge,
insert block.

C

Wedge removed.

Foot wedged into
dorsi-flexion.

D

Wedge closed.

Block.

E

Opened wedge
in cast.

a–shows uncut
lateral portion
of cast.

Lateral
angulation of
femur correc-
ted by wedging.

F

Fig. 23.—Technique of correcting angulation of fracture fragments by plaster cast wedging.

78

Correction of angulation by plaster cast wedging may be carried out if roentgenograms subsequent to the bone graft operation show persistent angulation. It must not be delayed until the callus begins to consolidate (Fig. 23).

The graft may be obtained from the same bone provided it is adequate in size and one of the fragments is sufficiently long and not too weak from disuse atrophy. Often, however, it is prefer-

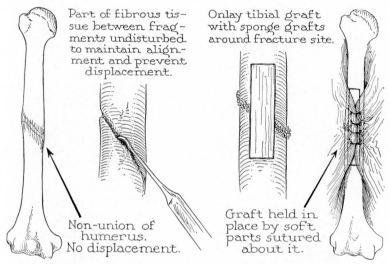

Part of fibrous tissue between fragments undisturbed to maintain alignment and prevent displacement.

Non-union of humerus. No displacement.

Onlay tibial graft with sponge grafts around fracture site.

Graft held in place by soft parts sutured about it.

Fig. 24.—Treatment of nonunion with an onlay bone graft.

able to obtain bone from some other location. The tibia is ordinarily used because of its length, density and easy accessibility. Iliac bone or refrigerated bone from a bone bank is preferable under some circumstances.

The following procedure is recommended for treating nonunion of the shaft of one of the long bones.

TREATMENT OF NONUNION OF LONG BONES

1. Use general or regional anesthesia.
2. Expose the site of the fracture.

3. Obtain accurate realignment of the fracture fragments. The fibrous tissue between the bone ends should be removed when necessary for adequate reduction.

4. If the ends of the fragments are hard and sclerotic, they should be perforated by means of a drill introduced in

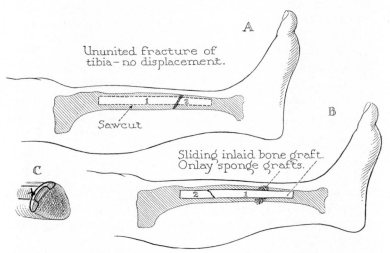

Fig. 25.—Technique of the autogenous inlay bone graft operation. The bone graft is reversed in its position. The term "sliding graft" is not appropriate, although it is widely used.

multiple areas and directions, leaving the bone powder in situ.

5. Using a broad chisel, prepare a flat surface, on which to apply the bone graft, extending across the fracture line.

6. A full thickness tibial bone graft with the cancellous side against the shaft of the fracture fragments is so placed that it crosses the fracture site for a distance adequate to get contact with healthy bone of each fragment, 2 to 4 in. on each side.

7. Place around the fracture site additional cancellous bone obtained from the same location as was the large graft.

If the nonunion is in a large bone such as the tibia or femur of an adult, it is wise to use two or more massive grafts, placed on opposite surfaces of the bone.

8. After the grafts have been placed and the incision closed, apply an adequate plaster dressing while the fragments are held accurately aligned and supported on the fracture table (Fig. 24).

In some cases it will be advisable to pass two threaded pins transversely through each fragment at some distance above and below the fracture site. The ends of these wires should be incorporated in the plaster cast, leaving the adjacent joints free. This will allow the patient to be ambulatory. This joint freedom may be definitely indicated if there has been a prolonged period of immobilization during earlier treatment.

Sliding inlay bone grafts are frequently used in nonunion of fractures of the tibia. The technique is shown in Figure 25. This operation is highly successful unless the tibia is exceedingly atrophic, in which case the graft should be obtained from the uninjured tibia, ilium or bone bank.

CHAPTER XIII

Complications of Fractures

IN addition to loss of continuity of bone, a fracture may produce or be attended by injuries to nerves, blood vessels, muscles, tendons or joints. Some complications are immediate, while others are secondary and remote, affecting organs or tissues far removed from the site of the local trauma. These complications or sequelae may include one or more of the following conditions:

1. Shock
   a) Primary
   b) Secondary
2. Fat embolism
3. Pneumonia
4. Injuries to the central or peripheral nervous system
   a) Acute or immediate
      (1) Compression or severance of a peripheral nerve
      (2) Concussion of the spinal cord (see Chapter **XXX**)
      (3) Concussion of the brain (see Chapter **XXXIII**)
      (4) Transection of the spinal cord (see Chapter **XXX**)

      b) Delayed complications
- (1) Secondary neuritis
- (2) Late palsy

5. Injury to the urinary bladder or urethra (see Chapter **XXXI**)
6. Volkmann's paralysis
7. Infection
8. Rupture of tendons
9. Acute atrophy of bone
10. Subperiosteal or ligamentous ossification
11. Arrest of growth of the bone that is fractured
12. Gangrene
13. Pressure sores
14. Renal calculi
15. Malunion
16. Traumatic arthritis

SHOCK.—The most serious of all fracture complications, because it holds the most immediate threat of death, is that known as *traumatic shock.* The subject will be discussed under two divisions: primary shock, and secondary or wound shock.

Primary shock is a neurocirculatory phenomenon. It is probably caused by a reflex splanchnic dilatation with concomitant cerebral anemia. Mild shock is similar in many respects to simple syncope. If there is no other more serious reason for shock, the patient will recover promptly when treated in the recumbent position by the application of external heat, the relief of pain and the administration of a stimulant such as ammonia vapor (to be inhaled).

Secondary or wound shock is much more serious. It is the result of loss of blood or plasma. Blood may escape from the body through open wounds, or hemorrhage may occur into extensively contused muscles of an extremity or into a body cavity. If the fluid loss is extensive, shock may develop quickly, but more often it comes on insidiously and, if not combated, may cause death.

The appearance of the patient in a state of shock is typical and diagnostic. He may be entirely conscious and mentally alert, but he will be exceedingly weak and apprehensive. The surface of the body is cold and often moist. There are pallor of the lips and cheeks and cyanosis of the nails, ears and mucous membranes. The pulse is thready and rapid. Intense thirst may be present.

Treatment of either primary or secondary shock should always precede or accompany débridement of a wound or attempts at closed reduction of a fracture. The immediate treatment is outlined below.

IMMEDIATE TREATMENT OF SHOCK

1. Exclude cerebral concussion as a cause of the patient's symptoms.
2. Arrest the hemorrhage by
   a) Pressure over, or packing of, the wound,
   b) Application of a tourniquet *just long enough* to prepare the wound for isolation of major bleeding blood vessels.
3. Splint the injured limb immediately—to prevent local loss of tissue fluids and pain due to movement of the ends of the fractured bone.
4. Provide heat; keep the patient surrounded with warm blankets.
5. Raise the foot of the bed or stretcher.
6. Give the patient hot tea or coffee, *except* when
   a) The patient is unconscious, and
   b) There are abdominal wounds with possible injury to the stomach or intestines, or
   c) A general anesthetic is contemplated.

7. Administer morphine, gr. ¼, to relieve pain and restlessness.
8. Administer oxygen.
9. Give massive transfusions of blood or plasma, or both.
10. The restoration to normal of the blood concentration may be ascertained by hematocrit determination.

Control of hemorrhage, restoration of body warmth, relief of pain and the replacement of blood by intravenous injection of 2 to 4 pt. of whole blood or human plasma will relieve the shock and save the life of many patients who otherwise would have been doomed at the outset. Blood plasma or serum should be given slowly and continuously during the operation of débridement. If ample amounts of these substances are not available, intravenous injection of 5 per cent glucose and normal saline should be given and continued for some hours thereafter. Administration of oxygen in high concentration should be continued as long as cyanosis of the lips, ears or nails persists.

FAT EMBOLISM is one of three fracture complications which may cause sudden death. Records indicate that it is at least a contributory factor in many of the deaths which follow fracture injuries. When fat from the bone marrow enters the blood stream, the larger droplets are filtered out in the lungs, while those which pass through the pulmonary capillaries scatter throughout the body. The symptoms may be those of acute edema of the lungs, with dyspnea, cyanosis, precordial pain, cough, hyperpyrexia and (occasionally) delirium due to cerebral irritation. The diagnosis may be confirmed by demonstrating the presence of fat in the urine and sputum. Fortunately, most cases are mild and the patients recover. When there are marked signs of cerebral irritation with tremor or stupor, death usually results. Fat embolism is less common when the surgeon insists on early and complete immobilization with the least possible amount of manipulation for his patients.

PNEUMONIA has been a common complication following major fractures in elderly individuals. Usually it is the result of hypostatic congestion of the lungs, produced by the recumbent position of the patient whose circulation is already impaired. Early ambulation is the best method of preventing hypostatic pneumonia. If possible, get the patient out of bed, either on crutches or into a wheel chair. Regular turning from side to side or from back to abdomen every six hours (or at least twice every 24 hours) should be carried out by the nurses. Whenever possible, this procedure should be supervised by the attending surgeon or a member of the resident staff. Continuous elevation of the head of the bed, or of the patient's head and shoulders by means of pillows, is thought to be of some value. The lungs should be frequently checked for the development of edema or consolidation. At the first sign of either, penicillin in adequate doses should be given.

INJURIES TO PERIPHERAL NERVES.—Peripheral nerves may be injured at the time of the fracture or during treatment by open reduction or manipulation. For his own protection as well as that of his patients, the physician should make a careful neurologic examination to determine before operation whether or not a nerve lesion has been produced by the injury. The neurologic findings should be recorded in the history. If, for example, a radial nerve palsy is present and is not brought to the attention of the patient or his family before a manipulation or open reduction of the fracture is performed, the physician may be unable to prove that he is not responsible for the lesion. Prognosis and treatment are also intimately related to the time of onset of the nerve injury.

Acute nerve palsy follows immediately or occurs within a few days after the fracture and may result from contusion, compression, stretching or laceration of a peripheral nerve or nerve root. The symptoms vary from those of pain to numbness and complete paralysis of the muscles. Acute neuritis or palsy occurs most often in the ulnar, musculospiral, peroneal (more often compressed by a poorly applied splint or cast, the edge of which falls just back of the head of the fibula) and sciatic nerves (as a complication of posterior dislocation of the hip). Muscles para-

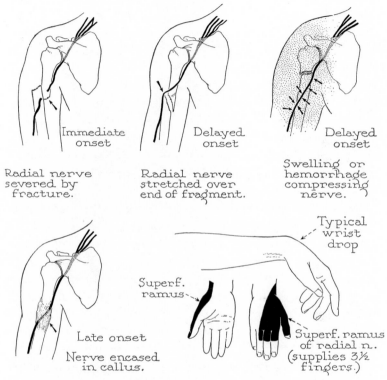

Fig. 26.—Injuries to the musculospiral nerve which may complicate fractures of the humerus.

lyzed as a result of nerve injuries must be supported by an adequate splint in a position of physiologic rest which shortens and relaxes the muscle fibers. Acute palsy is often temporary. Recovery may follow reduction and immobilization of the fracture or relief of pressure from a cast or splint. If there are no signs of recovery after six to 10 weeks, complete severance of the nerve may be assumed, and exploration with nerve repair is indicated (Figs. 26 and 27).

Secondary neuritis, manifested by pain, loss of function or

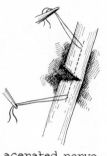

Lacerated nerve.
Orientation sutures
placed in nerve sheath.

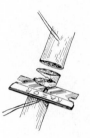

Laceration
excised

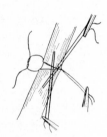

Stay sutures on
each side.

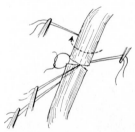

Nerve turned by traction on stay
sutures to expose front and back.
Sutures only thru nerve sheath.

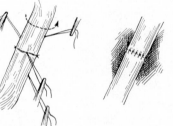

Completed suture.
Orientation sutures
removed.

FIG. 27.—A lacerated nerve must be accurately repaired after careful excision of the damaged portion.

both, may be caused by overproduction of callus or fibrous tissue which surrounds and compresses the nerve during the healing of the fracture. Characteristically, the symptoms come on late and progress as the fracture heals. Surgery is indicated for the purpose of neurolysis.

Late nerve palsy may appear many years after a fracture. By far the most common form of this complication is late ulnar nerve palsy. This results from a fracture of the elbow with non-union, malunion or growth arrest of the lateral condyle. A cubitus valgus deformity may develop by continued growth of the medial condyle of the humerus. The ulnar nerve is stretched by motion of the elbow, and a neuroma may form where the nerve trunk passes behind the medial epicondyle. This is best treated by transplantation of the nerve to a position anterior to the condyle. The deformity may be corrected by an osteotomy of the lower end of the humerus.

VOLKMANN'S PARALYSIS (often called ischemic paralysis) is a misnomer for a condition produced by compression of the veins while the arteries continue to carry blood into the extremity. The occlusion of the veins may be due to pressure from fracture fragments, a cast or splint that is too tight or acute edema or hemorrhage beneath the deep fascia. Probably the last is the most frequent cause. The deep fascia is nonelastic, and subfascial pressure may be so great that all veins are collapsed, but not sufficient to compress the arteries. Volkmann's deformity occurs most often in the forearm following a fracture in the region of the elbow. Severe pain in the forearm or in the lower leg after a crushing injury in the region just below the elbow or just distal to the knee, associated with swelling of the extremity and cyanosis of the fingers or toes, should be accepted as a warning of a developing Volkmann contracture. The *cast or splint on such an extremity should be removed at once, the part elevated and a sympathetic nerve block performed.* If circulation does not improve, the deep fascia should be exposed and widely opened to facilitate the escape of fluids and reduce the subfascial pressure. If the pressure is not reduced soon after the symptoms appear, severe and permanent damage will result. This includes disruption of nerve and muscle cells and replacement by dense fibrous tissue. Contractures follow, with the development of a badly deformed and frequently a functionally useless hand or leg.

Watson-Jones describes another type of severe disability quite similar to Volkmann's contracture which he considers to be the result of *brachial artery contusion* with resulting arterial spasm. This is associated with paralysis of the limb, while in Volkmann's contracture the involvement of sensory nerves or of motor fibers themselves is minimal or entirely absent. What Volkmann really described was the contracture of the muscles due to fibrosis. It now appears evident that the deformity can be produced by: (1) major artery spasm or rupture; (2) venous obstruction from internal or external pressure.

INFECTION, whether the result of contamination of an open fracture or of an open reduction of a closed fracture, may lead to *osteomyelitis* with delayed union or nonunion and loss of varying amounts of bone substance through sequestration. The treatment of open or infected fractures has been discussed in Chapter XI.

TENDONS MAY BE RUPTURED or severed at the time of the injury, or they may tear apart after the fracture has healed. Severe contusion of a tendon at the time of the initial injury may result, 14–21 days later, in rupture due to softening and necrosis of the tendon fibers. Usually, however, a delayed rupture is caused by constant irritation produced by repeated movement of the tendon back and forth over a projecting rough or sharp bone splinter or callus after function is resumed. The ruptured tendon, whether developing acute or late, should be sutured as soon as the condition is diagnosed.

ACUTE ATROPHY OF BONE is infrequent but does occur. This was described by Sudeck, who called it "post-traumatic acute bone atrophy." The condition is associated with pain, loss of function of the entire extremity, edema and marked decalcification of the bone. The skin becomes shiny and trophic. As with most atrophy of bone and swelling of soft parts produced by disuse and inactivity, the responsibility for occurrence of this condition rests, as a rule, with the surgeon. Acute atrophy of bone usually means that during the period of immobilization of the fracture the surgeon has failed properly to emphasize to

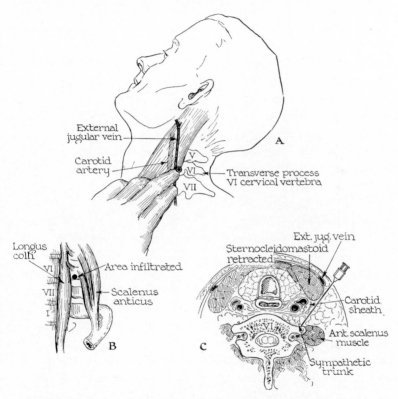

External jugular vein

Carotid artery

V

VI

VII

Transverse process VI cervical vertebra

A

Longus colli'

VI

VII

I

Area infiltrated

Scalenus anticus

B

Ext. jug. vein

Sternocleidomastoid retracted

Carotid sheath

Ant. scalenus muscle

Sympathetic trunk

VI

C

FIG. 28.—Technique for procaine injection of the cervical sympathetics in treatment of painful neurovascular conditions in the upper extremity, such as the distressing syndromes sometimes designated as causalgia or Sudeck's atrophy of bone with pain and edema. *A,* after J. A. Caldwell.

the patient the importance of functional activity of all joints, to the fullest extent possible. Acute atrophy, fibrous adhesions of tendons and muscles and accompanying loss of function can be prevented if the patient is compelled to co-operate from the very beginning by actively, vigorously and frequently contracting all of the muscles of the immobilized extremity. (See Figs. 28 and 29.)

SUBPERIOSTEAL OR LIGAMENTOUS OSSIFICATION may occur

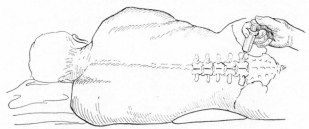

A Skin wheals for lumbar plexus block.

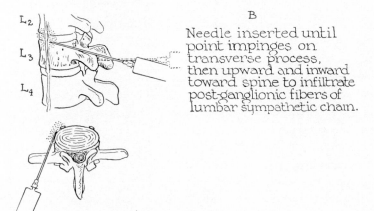

B
Needle inserted until point impinges on transverse process, then upward and inward toward spine to infiltrate post-ganglionic fibers of lumbar sympathetic chain.

FIG. 29.—A technique for lumbar sympathetic block by procaine should be mastered by every fracture surgeon. The value of this treatment has been well established in relief of vasospasm and impending gangrene following crushing injuries to the lower extremities.

following fractures in the region of a joint. This is most common at the elbow. It is, in effect, a process similar to, if not identical with, the myositis ossificans traumatica which frequently occurs in subperiosteal hematomas, following severe bruising of muscles of the thigh and (more rarely) other portions of the extremities. We are of the opinion that traumatic ossification about joints is increased by forced movement and passive stretching, which continue to traumatize the injured tissues.

ARREST OF BONE GROWTH.—Fractures in children should sound the alert for one hazard peculiar to childhood. The growth center of every long bone is found in a cartilage plate which is located between the epiphysis and the diaphysis. On the diaphyseal side of the cartilage plate there are columns of cartilage cells which contribute to longitudinal growth. A crushing injury to this growth center, or a fracture of the shaft of the bone which crosses the epiphyseal cartilage plate and enters the epiphysis, may result in the formation of a bridge of bone which unites the epiphysis to the diaphysis. This, in effect, rigidly checks a part of or all further elongation of the shaft which should have occurred from that center of growth. If the patient is young and several growth years lie ahead, this will lead to a progressive deformity and relative shortening of the extremity. There is no certainty that the most accurate reduction will prevent growth arrest, and the prognosis should be guarded. Early accurate reduction and most careful immobilization must be insisted on whenever the fracture reaches or crosses the growth center zone. Children who have sustained such fractures should be re-examined, both clinically and by x-ray, at six month intervals until they have attained adult growth.

If growth arrest does occur, the deformity can be minimized through osteotomy; if the arrest is only partial, surgical closure of the growing side of the plate is indicated to prevent deformity of the adjacent joint. If the injury is in the tibia or distal end of the femur, surgical growth arrest should be produced in the corresponding epiphyseal plate of the opposite extremity to prevent inequality of leg length (Fig. 30).

GANGRENE occasionally follows a severe fracture. It may be the result of arterial injury from the sharp edges of the fracture fragments but can also result from unskilful application of a plaster cast which constricts the circulation. Gangrene of this type can be prevented by frequent inspection of circulation of the fingers or toes and by splitting the cast if these digits become cold or cyanotic. A safe plan is to split the plaster cast at the time it is applied, to permit it to spread as swelling within the cast increases.

Circulatory disturbances, other than acute arterial occlusion

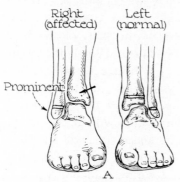
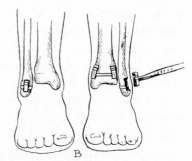

Right (affected)   Left (normal)

Prominent

A

Closure of distal tibial epiphysis on right following fracture with overgrowth of distal fibular epiphysis.

B

Treat by doing surgical arrest of fibular epiphysis on affected leg and of both tibial and fibular epiphyses on normal leg.

FIG. 30.—Treatment of deformity of the ankle caused by growth arrest of the tibia following a fracture which crossed the growth center and epiphysis.

leading to gangrene, may include the blistering of the skin which occasionally occurs as a sequel to marked swelling following a crushing injury. This complication is common in comminuted fractures of the os calcis. It can be prevented by supporting the circulation immediately after the injury and before the edema has become acute, with a properly applied *massive pressure dressing*.

When the circulation of the limb is seriously impaired, repeated sympathetic blocks as often as every four hours may produce dramatic improvement and prevent gangrene. If adequate circulation cannot be maintained by repeated satisfactory blocks, sympathectomy may be advisable.

PRESSURE SORES occur over bony prominences of patients who are elderly and emaciated. They are most common in patients who have suffered sensory loss because of injury of the spinal cord. These ulcers develop most often over the sacrum. Frequent turning of the patient and treatment of the back with tincture of benzoin or alcohol will usually prevent them.

Other bony prominences may be the site of pressure owing to inexpert application of plaster casts or to negligence in nursing care. Pressure sores are, in effect, trophic ulcers. They heal slowly. Treatment should consist of the excision of all necrotic tissue, use of a petrolatum pack and application of a closed plaster dressing. Meticulous care should be taken to prevent pressure on the ulcer from either the cast or the weight of the patient. Chemotherapy is of value during the acute phase in controlling secondary infection. Large skin defects are best treated by débridement and closure of the wound by the local shifting of skin and subcutaneous tissue.

RENAL CALCULI form very commonly in patients kept relatively inert in bed for many weeks or longer. This is attributed to inadequate drainage of the kidneys and the outpouring of calcium salts that occurs in disuse atrophy of the skeleton. Their formation may be prevented by:
1. An adequate fluid intake.
2. Maximal drainage of kidneys, insured by
    a) Frequent change of the patient's position in bed, with the trunk elevated.
    b) Ambulation (daily periods, if possible) to promote recovery of the atrophic bones through use and, at the same time, to facilitate postural drainage of the kidneys.

MALUNION may be considered a complication of a fracture

(Fig. 31). It may include marked over-riding with shortening of an extremity and angulation to a degree that interferes with or makes impossible satisfactory use of the part concerned. Before consolidation of the callus, malunion may sometimes be corrected by manipulation which achieves accurate reduction and align-

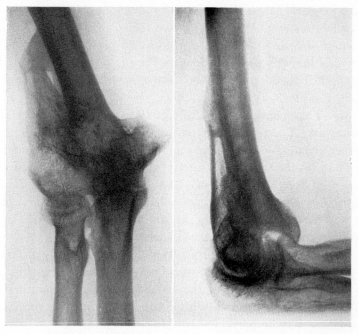

Fig. 31.—Malunion with almost complete ankylosis of the elbow following comminuted fracture of the condyles of the humerus.

ment. The fracture that is well healed in malposition can be corrected only by an open surgical procedure. In such fractures the bone fragments are separated with a chisel, and end-to-end apposition and good alignment are obtained. A cortical bone graft of full thickness may then be placed onlay or inlay across the line of osteotomy, to decrease the danger of nonunion in

bone fragments which may already have expended their osteogenetic force. Internal fixation of the graft and fracture fragments will insure maintenance of accurate reduction.

Many malunited fractures which could be corrected in adults
only by surgery may be treated conservatively in children because
of the ability of growing bones to compensate during subsequent
growth. In children, shortening of long bones as a result of fractures which healed with over-riding of as much as one-half inch
will usually catch up to or will grow beyond the corresponding
bone of the uninjured member as a result of epiphyseal stimula-
tion by the hyperemia associated with the repair of the defect.
Malunited fractures in the juxta-epiphyseal area of a long bone
must be treated with both skill and caution. Surgery in that
location may permanently arrest longitudinal growth. Surgical
correction of metaphyseal malunions should be delayed for at
least one year, during which time the deformity may correct
itself, or the zone of deformity, through growth of the bone, may
become farther removed from the growth cartilage so that the
operation can be performed with less risk. Corrections of angular
deformities of the midshaft of long bones seldom occur spontaneously, but surgery should be avoided unless function is definitely impaired.

TRAUMATIC ARTHRITIS may result when the fracture enters a
joint. This is more likely to occur if replacement of the fracture
fragments is not accurate. Atrophy of articular cartilage or
hypertrophic changes in joints may result from long-continued
push or pull forces. The well-leg traction splint is objectionable
because of this feature. Traumatic arthritis rarely occurs when
accurate reduction has been maintained, with the resumption of
functional activity as soon as union is firm.

CHAPTER XIV

Aseptic Necrosis of Bone

BONE is a hard substance which must withstand stresses and strains and support body weight. It is, however, living tissue and to remain viable must have an exchange of blood and lymph. Following any fracture, there is a varying degree of bone necrosis at the ends of the fragments because of rupture of the nutrient vessels or stripping of the periosteum, or both. If disruption of circulation is only partial, the bone fragments will usually live and union will follow reduction and immobilization. In other instances, portions of the bone may be isolated from their blood supply and, thus deprived of nutrition, will die. This process is called avascular or aseptic necrosis in contradistinction to septic necrosis, where loss of blood supply follows infection.

Aseptic necrosis is most frequently observed in the head of the femur after intracapsular fractures and traumatic dislocations of the hip (Fig. 32). Less frequently, it follows fractures of the base of the neck and intertrochanteric regions as well as chronic slipping of the proximal femoral epiphysis. Aseptic necrosis may be associated with a fracture of the carpal navicular, dislocation of the lunate, fracture of the astragalus or a comminuted or

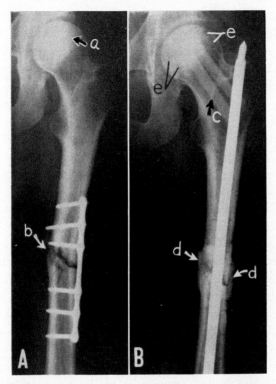

Fig. 32.—*A,* aseptic necrosis of the head of the femur, *a,* following dislocation of the hip and nonunion of a fracture of the shaft of the femur at the
juncture of the middle and proximal thirds, *b.* The fracture of the femur was
plated 2 weeks following the injury, and the dislocation of the hip was reduced by open operation 8 weeks after the injury. *B,* five months following
the injury, two tibial bone grafts, *c,* were placed through the neck of the
femur into the femoral head and the nonunion of the shaft of the femur was
treated at the same operation with an intramedullary rod introduced downward through the trochanter. Bone grafts were placed around the fracture
site, *d.* Advanced replacement of the femoral head by creeping substitution is
demonstrated, *e.* Protection from weight-bearing must be continued until this
replacement is completed.

99

segmental fracture of any bone when a fragment is deprived of its vascular connections.

Axhausen first described the pathology of aseptic necrosis, but our knowledge of this condition has been greatly enlarged by the careful studies of Phemister and his co-workers during the past 20 years. The microscopic changes in aseptic necrosis may be summarized thus:

The bone fragment, including cortex, trabeculae and marrow, becomes partially or totally necrotic. The articular cartilage, which may be a part of the fragment, will in some cases survive to a varying degree.

The cancellous spaces of the bone are spontaneously invaded by a vascularized connective tissue which reaches the fragment through adhesions or from the adjacent living bone as union is established. This invasion proceeds in a centrifugal fashion so as to establish vascular connections with all portions of the fragment. While the process may continue to completion, it may be arrested and leave areas of varying size uninvaded and unreplaced. The dead marrow is first replaced by fibrous tissue but eventually fatty or hemapoietic marrow appears.

The necrotic bone (trabeculae and articular cortex) may be completely absorbed in some areas producing temporary fibrous zones. When new trabeculae do appear in these fibrous zones, meager amounts of bone may be formed, leaving the head more or less fibrous. The dead trabeculae may also be transformed into living bone while they are undergoing absorption. Osteoblasts reappear on their surfaces and viability returns by gradual restitution. Devitalized bone can be microscopically distinguished by its poor staining properties and the absence of osteoblasts on the surface and in the lacunae.

Revascularization of a dead femoral head is an orderly process (Fig. 33). First there is invasion by fibrous tissue which brings in a new blood supply *(zone of invasion)*. The first invaded area will soon show regions where dead bone has diminished *(zone of absorption)*. As the zone of invasion moves further into the head, it is followed by the zone of absorption. The oldest region of invasion and first zone of absorption will now show evidence of new bone formation and this is called the *zone of restitution*. When the zone of absorption approaches the periphery, the bony articular cortex is absorbed along with the subcortical bone. Articular cartilage, however, gets a portion of its nutriment from the synovial fluid and, while it will survive in children under 10,

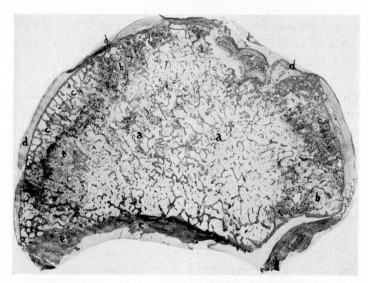

Fig. 33.—Section through the head of a femur which has undergone aseptic necrosis: *a*, fine trabeculae of new bone; *b*, advancing zone of fibrous tissue; *c*, dead bone which is being absorbed where it is in contact with the fibrous tissue; *d*, old hyaline articular cartilage which is also undergoing degenerative changes; *e*, sclerotic bone in the line of the ununited fracture. This indicates that there was motion and friction between the contacting fracture surfaces. (Courtesy of Dr. C. H. Hatcher.)

it will rarely remain viable in the adolescent child or adult. When hyaline cartilage dies and is absorbed, it is replaced by fibrous connective tissue or fibrocartilage.

Frequently osteo-arthritis is superimposed on the necrotic articular bone. It is characterized pathologically by a villous synovitis, sclerosis or eburnation of the opposed contacting bone, osteophyte formation at the articular margins and, occasionally, the formation of loose bodies in the joint. The severity of the arthritis depends on the degree of preservation of the shape of the rejuvenated femoral head. Arthritis is most marked if the head breaks up into fragments, as it does when unprotected weight-bearing is permitted before repair is complete.

The DIAGNOSIS of a dead femoral head can be made by microscopic or roentgen examination. Rarely is tissue available for histologic preparations during the treatment of acute injury and we depend on roentgenograms not only for early diagnosis but also for following the reparative process. Roentgen diagnosis is considered under two headings, *early* and *late*.

The *early roentgen diagnosis* of a necrotic femoral head is based on changes in the living bone at the *proximal end of the femur and acetabulum* but not in the head itself. Since the head is separated from its blood vessels at the time of the accident, the constituents of the fragment will remain inert and unchanged until blood supply is gradually restored. This requires many months to become demonstrable in roentgenograms and several years to complete. A roentgenogram of the dead head during the first two to four months will ordinarily show no changes. The density of the bone will remain the same as at the time of the accident. The trabecular pattern is normal and the joint space is not ordinarily narrowed. The living bone of the proximal femur and acetabulum will, in such instances, undergo atrophy of disuse since the patient is unable to use the extremity during the periods of immobilization and protection from weight-bearing necessary for healing the fracture. The contrast between the dead femoral head which *has retained its original density* and the surrounding living bone which has undergone atrophy of disuse can be demonstrated on good roentgenograms and, although the diagnosis cannot be established until two to four months following the injury, it is referred to as the *early diagnosis* of a dead femoral head.

Late diagnosis depends, on the other hand, on alterations within the head itself. They consist of changes in *contour,* as seen after fracture or multiple fracture of the dead bone from walking on it, or changes in the trabecular pattern, articular cortex or narrowing of the joint spaces as invasion and replacement take place. The irregular absorption of necrotic bone and the formation of new atrophic living bone produce the irregular mottled roentgen appearance so characteristic of the replacement stage. The progressive rejuvenation of the fragment can be followed on serial roentgenograms as more and more of the bone becomes mottled and irregularly reduced in density, while the shadow of articular cortex disappears only to re-form somewhat with time. Finally, the joint space will show narrowing as fibrocartilage replaces articular hyaline cartilage. Accurate interpretation of the progressive roentgen changes in terms of the microhistologic process enables the physician to plan intelligently the treatment of his patient.

Nonunions commonly occur when a fracture fragment becomes necrotic. On the other hand, union may occur between the dead and the living fragments. In a nonweight-bearing bone, such as the navicular or lunate, the dead fragment may undergo satisfactory progressive restitution as blood vessels cross the site of union. If the necrotic fragment is in the lower extremity, it must be recognized early and protected in walking by the use of crutches. If unprotected, the dead bone or the fragile regenerated bone will collapse from the superincumbent weight of the body. In the hip, new fractures are prone to occur across the head of the femur through the junction of the unreplaced and transformed portions. If, on the other hand, the head is adequately protected from weight-bearing until roentgenograms show complete restitution of the dead bone, the prognosis is hopeful and the patient may be rewarded with a good hip.

Occasionally a dead femoral head may unite with the shaft and stand up under weight-bearing for several years before it collapses. The patient will then return complaining of pain, muscle spasm and a limp. The clinical diagnosis would suggest traumatic osteo-arthritis. There is a difference of opinion, among those who have studied the problem of late collapse of the femoral head after union has taken place, as to the time of onset of the necrosis—whether it begins *immediately* after the accident or *after several years* of the trauma of normal function. While the immediate fate of the head of the femur appears to be determined by the extent of the disruption of its circulation at the time of the fracture, one of us (E.L.C.) has suggested that delayed necrosis may occur in a head which remained viable after the fracture but lacked sufficient vitality to survive the repeated minimal traumas exerted on it by motion, muscle action and weight-bearing of everyday activity.

ASEPTIC NECROSIS OF THE HEAD OF FEMUR AFTER INTRA-CAPSULAR FRACTURES.—*The blood supply of the head of the femur* in the adult is derived from the arteries of the round ligament and from the nutrient branches of the anterior and posterior circumflex femoral arteries which enter the epiphysis after passing through the capsule on the neck and the retinacula, especially the one most posteriorly placed (Fig. 138). The vessels which enter by way of the capsule are generally regarded as the more important, although Chandler and Kreuscher, Wolcott, Nordenson and others have shown by anatomic studies that arteries are present in the round ligament and are of significant size in most hips of all ages. Conclusive evidence is lacking as to exactly which of the aforementioned vessels are most important in maintaining the circulation of the head of the femur.

In intracapsular fractures of the femur, with separation of the fragments, the blood vessels which pass along the neck are torn to a greater or less degree. If the blood supply of the remaining capsular vessels, together with that of the round ligament, is inadequate to maintain nutrition of the head, the head of the femur will undergo necrosis.

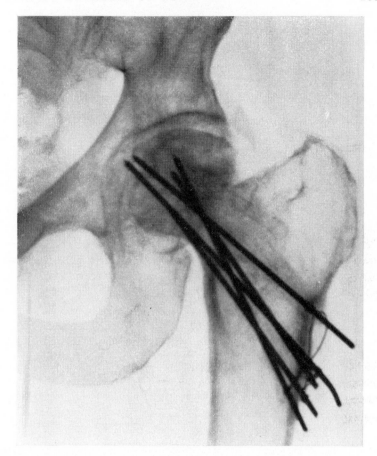

FIG. 34.—Aseptic necrosis of head of the femur with beginning collapse of the portion of cortex bearing most weight stress. See also Figure 35.

The possibility of the head of the femur undergoing aseptic necrosis and the important role it plays in the final functional result should be kept in mind by the surgeon who undertakes the care of fractures of the femoral neck. He must reduce the fracture with the least possible amount of additional trauma, main-

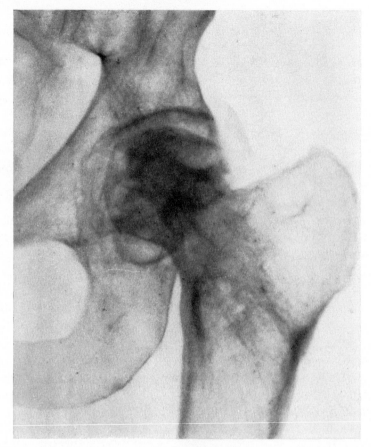

Fig. 35.—Same case as preceding. Union of the fracture followed open reduction, tibial bone graft and threaded pin fixation. The femoral head shows advanced but incomplete replacement.

tain reduction of the fracture with internal fixation, protect the hip from weight-bearing to permit union to take place and determine as soon as possible by roentgenograms whether the head is dead or alive. If the head becomes necrotic, protection of the hip by means of crutches, so that no weight will be borne by the extremity, should be prolonged until there is roentgen evidence of complete restitution of the dead bone. Restitution can be hastened, as shown by Phemister, by the insertion of two tibial bone grafts into the head through a lateral incision (Figs. 32, 34 and 35). When the state of necrosis is not recognized and walking is resumed, collapse and fragmentation of the head are likely to occur (Fig. 36). Fracture of the neck of the femur with dislocation of the femoral head disrupts the blood supply to the head so completely that one may anticipate death of the proximal fragment in practically all such cases. The treatment of aseptic necrosis of the femoral head without union of the fracture is described in Chapter XXIV.

Intertrochanteric fractures occasionally tear the anterior or the posterior circumflex vessel, or both, with secondary necrosis of the proximal portion of the neck and the entire head.

Traumatic dislocations of the hip are followed in a large percentage of cases by late return of pain in the hip, with clinical and roentgenologic evidence of osteo-arthritis of this joint. Formerly these poor end-results were merely labeled traumatic arthritis. They are now recognized to be late manifestations of aseptic necrosis of the femoral head, secondary to the tearing of blood vessels at the time of the original injury. Because of the high incidence of necrosis, the following procedure is recommended.

Whenever possible, the extremity should be protected from weight-bearing by use of crutches for four to six months after the postreduction period of immobilization or recumbency; this is for diagnosis only, and not the prevention of necrosis. *Necrosis occurs from loss of blood supply.* If the femoral head undergoes uniform atrophy of disuse and after six months its density does not differ from that of the then osteoporotic living bone of the femoral shaft and of the ilium as shown roentgenographically, the patient may resume full weight-bearing with the likelihood that the head has remained alive. Roentgenographic follow-ups

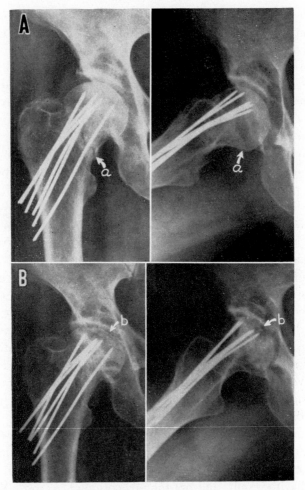

Fig. 36.—*A*, healed subcapital fracture of the neck of the femur, with clinically normal function. *a*, line of fracture still visible. *B*, same patient four years later, revealing breakdown in the cortex of the femoral head, *b*, probably as a result of aseptic necrosis with creeping replacement. The presence of necrosis of the femoral head was not recognized in the earlier films.

at three month intervals should be continued for an additional 12 months. If, however, the head is necrotic it should be removed and replaced by a plastic or metallic prosthesis.

ASEPTIC NECROSIS OF THE CARPAL SCAPHOID AND LUNATE BONES.—In the upper extremity the carpal *scaphoid* is the bone most often injured as a result of disruption of its blood supply, and in the incidence of avascular necrosis it is second only to the

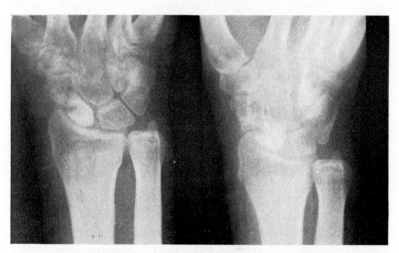

FIG. 37.—Ununited fracture of the scaphoid bone of the wrist with aseptic necrosis of the proximal fragment. Note the contrast in density between the living atrophic and the necrotic unchanged portion of the bone.

head of the femur. Fractures through the waist of the carpal scaphoid result in necrosis of the proximal fragment in about one third of all cases. Following at least six weeks' immobilization, roentgenograms will show atrophy of the living distal fragment and the other carpal bones, while the proximal fragment cannot undergo atrophy. This contrast in relative density is diagnostic of necrosis of the proximal fragment (Fig. 37). Excision of the proximal or dead fragment, together with the radial styloid process (styloidectomy), is usually the treatment of choice. Loss of this fragment, even though osteo-arthritis has not developed, produces minimal alteration in the function of the wrist. An attempt to obtain union by drilling and peg bone grafts is not recommended when necrosis of a fragment is obvious. If the patient is engaged in manual labor, secondary arthritis of the radial-scaphoid and intercarpal articulations will inevitably develop and only an arthrodesis will offer relief. If the major portion of the scaphoid is necrotic the removal of both fragments, together with the lunate bone, and the radial-styloid process may be advisable. Precautionary measures should be taken in the operating room to insure excision of the desired fragment or fragments. *The exposed fragment should be marked with a needle or skin clip and a roentgenogram taken before the bone is removed.* This protects both the patient and the surgeon from the consequences of an irreparable error.

The carpal *lunate* bone frequently undergoes necrosis after anterior dislocation, even when reduction is promptly obtained. Open reduction in these cases is attended by an extremely high incidence of necrosis; the procedure should be avoided in recent injuries if possible. In old cases the bone should be excised.

ASEPTIC NECROSIS OF THE ASTRAGALUS.—Large nutrient blood vessels of the astragalus enter the bone on the anterolateral surface of the neck. Fractures through the neck of the astragalus may isolate the body of the bone from its major source of blood and, when the vessels entering by way of soft tissue attachments are not adequate to maintain viability, the body of the astragalus will undergo aseptic necrosis. Backward dislocation of the body of the astragalus associated with a fracture of the neck is almost always followed by necrosis.

The diagnosis is dependent on the roentgen features previously described, or on late pain in the ankle secondary to superimposed arthritis. If the astragalus collapses from weight-bearing and the ankle joint is disrupted, an arthrodesis of the astragalus to the tibia is indicated.

ASEPTIC NECROSIS OF OTHER BONES.—Necrosis due to a disruption of blood supply may occur in any bone following trauma sufficient to strip most of the soft tissue attachments and disrupt nutrient vessels. Typical findings of avascular necrosis may follow segmental fractures of the tibia or femur and some displaced fractures of the condyles of the femur or tibia.

CHAPTER XV

Pathologic Fractures

A FRACTURE may be correctly designated as pathologic if it occurs without a specific history of injury or as a result of minor trauma in a bone which has been weakened by a pre-existing disease or metabolic condition. Under this heading might be included fractures that occur as a result of trophic disturbances; for example, in neurotrophic joints (Fig. 38). Other constitutional and metabolic disturbances predisposing to fracture from minimal traumas are: rickets, osteomalacia, congenital fragility of bone (Fig. 39); senile osteoporosis, Paget's disease, multiple myeloma and generalized osteitis fibrosa. Local bone lesions which may predispose to fractures include: osteomyelitis, solitary bone cysts (Fig. 40), giant cell tumors and either primary or metastatic malignant growths (Figs. 41, 42 and 43). Deep x-ray therapy over the pelvis causes changes that have resulted in pathologic fracture of the femoral neck.

Fractures that are secondary to constitutional disturbances must be treated locally by an adequate reduction and proper immobilization while suitable therapy is administered for the disease. Rickets, osteomalacia and, to some extent, senile osteoporosis will respond favorably to the administration of vitamin D and a diet high in calcium. Fractures that occur secondary to tabes dorsalis and syringomyelia do not respond favorably to any type of therapy. The prognosis for healing of fractures which are secondary to a primary or metastatic malignant lesion is no better than that of the malignancy itself. Contrary to a com-

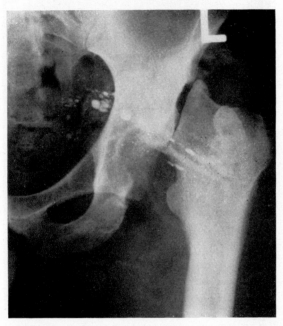

Fig. 38.—Pathologic fracture dislocation of the hip in a patient with tertiary syphilis. This fracture dislocation occurred spontaneously and was characteristically free from pain. Bismuth or other antisyphilitic medication is visible in the gluteus muscles.

monly expressed opinion, exceedingly atrophic bones, as for example in flail extremities after infantile paralysis, in which there is no specific local pathologic process, will heal as promptly as do normal bones following fracture. The strength of the union, however, will be relatively no greater than the strength of the bone fractured.

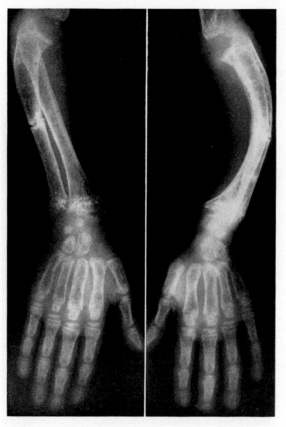

Fig. 39.—Osteogenesis imperfecta tarda with spontaneous fractures of forearm bones.

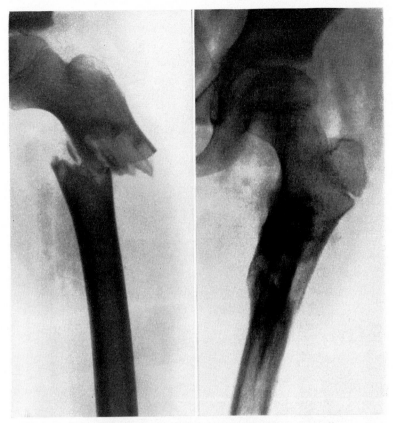

FIG. 40.—*Left,* pathologic fracture of femur through a large solitary bone cyst. *Right,* union after curettement of the cyst and insertion of a tibial bone graft.

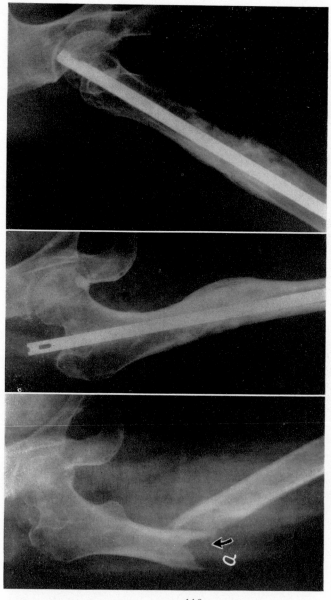

Fig. 41.—Pathologic fracture at the junction of the middle and proximal thirds of the femur through a metastatic lesion from carcinoma of the breast. The break is irregular and the proximal fragment shows destruction of the cortex, a. Intramedullary fixation of this type of fracture is the treatment of choice. Relief from pain and healing of the fracture will usually follow this immobilization.

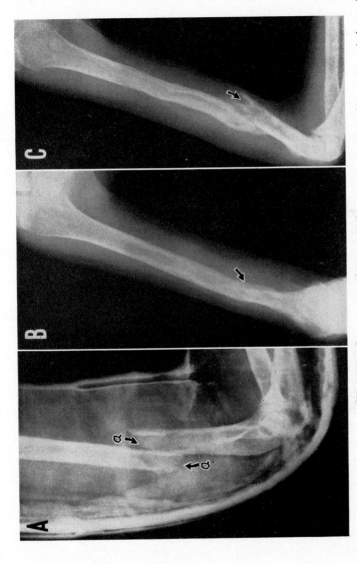

Fig. 42.—Pathologic fracture of the humerus of a patient with widespread skeletal lymphosarcoma. *A* shows the lytic lesions in each fragment. *a*. Immobilization in a snug-hanging cast surprisingly resulted in solid bone union, *B* and *C*, without x-ray or other therapy.

117

Pathologic fractures are treated by the same general principles and methods described for the various bones of the skeleton. Union can be attained in most instances. It is a mistake to with-

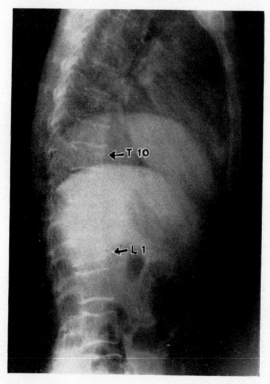

Fig. 43.—Spontaneous collapse of first lumbar vertebra and less marked collapse of tenth thoracic vertebra in a patient with widely disseminated multiple myeloma. The marked generalized appearance of osteoporosis is typical of this disease.

hold an open reduction or internal fixation because the patient may have an advanced malignancy. The remaining months of life of these patients should be spent at home with their families instead of in a hospital, even though this may require a major surgical procedure such as the insertion of an intramedullary rod, or any other form of internal fixation, which will permit ambulation on crutches.

CHAPTER XVI

Birth Fractures

FRACTURE of the shaft of the *humerus* is the commonest bone injury which occurs as a result of the handling of the infant during obstetric delivery. This occurs most often in breech deliveries during attempts to deliver the extended arms. The fracture may be either transverse or spiral; rarely is there any significant displacement. The deformity is readily recognized and the presence of fracture confirmed by roentgenologic examination. Treatment consists of strapping the arm to the side of the chest with a soft cotton or wool pad in the axilla. If angulation persists after union occurs, growth and remodeling of the bone will correct the dis-alignment. Traction may be utilized if necessary, as shown in Figure 101.

Fractures of the shaft of the *femur* and of the *clavicle* also occur in breech deliveries. A fracture of the clavicle is suggested if the baby fails to move one arm or cries when it is handled by the nurse or mother. Often this fracture is misdiagnosed because the symptoms are similar to those of brachial plexus palsy. Fracture of the clavicle, or the less common dislocation of either end of the clavicle, can be successfully treated by placing a soft rolled or elastic bandage as a figure-of-eight dressing of soft

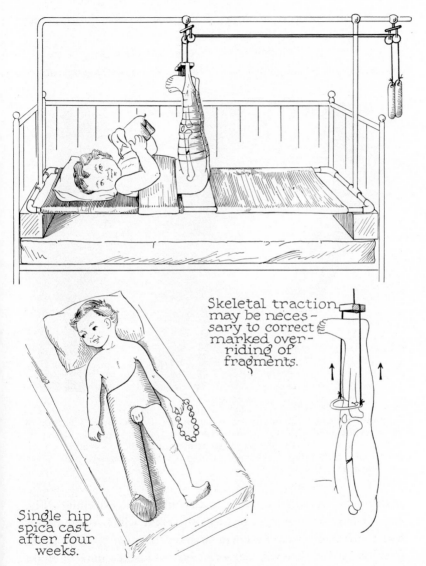

Skeletal traction may be necessary to correct marked overriding of fragments.

Single hip spica cast after four weeks.

FIG. 44.—Femoral fractures in infants and young children.

material around the shoulders. It may be necessary to bandage the involved arm to the trunk.

The fractured femur is readily recognized. It should be treated by means of overhead traction, with adhesive extension applied

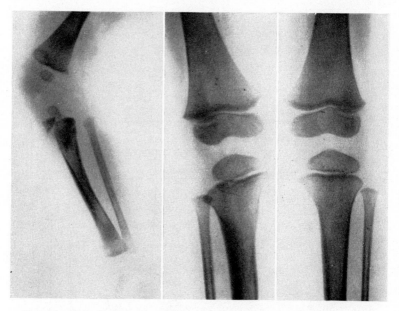

Fig. 45.—*Left,* birth injury which occurred during a breech delivery. The fracture fragment from the proximal end of the tibia included a portion of the growth center. *Center,* at the age of 2 years and 1 month the deformity is minimal. The growth cartilage plate is intact and there is reason to hope for complete restoration. *Right,* roentgenogram of the uninjured tibia shown for comparison.

both to the fractured leg and to the uninjured extremity (Fig. 44). If only one leg is suspended, the child will twist and turn and the fracture may heal with marked rotation or torsion deformity. Angulation will be corrected by further bone growth, but torsion may persist throughout life and should be prevented. An open reduction is rarely indicated.

CONGENITAL OSTEOGENESIS IMPERFECTA (also called fragilitas ossium or osteopsathyrosis) may result in multiple intrauterine fractures, some of which will have healed by the time of birth; other fractures are produced during the process of birth. When there are multiple fractures prior to or at the time of birth, with congenital fragility of bone, the infant rarely survives. In the milder form of fragilitas ossium, fractures may not be present at the time of birth but are prone to occur following slight injuries throughout infancy and childhood. This tendency to fracture becomes less as the child grows older, and after puberty the bones may be normal in strength.

There has been no satisfactory treatment for the infant born with multiple fractures. Glandular substances and vitamins have been employed as adjuncts to the immobilization of the fractures themselves, but their value has not been demonstrated.

BIRTH FRACTURES OF NORMAL BONES rarely include *epiphyseal displacements*. In most instances they are torsion fractures in the shaft at a distance from the growth centers. Occasionally an injury may result in wide stripping of periosteum, with subsequent aseptic necrosis of a considerable portion of a shaft of the femur or tibia. This may result in growth arrest, with subsequent shortening and deformity (Fig. 45).

CONGENITAL PSEUDARTHROSIS of the tibia may be present at birth or may appear during infancy as a result of congenital deficiencies in the tibia which lead to progressive bowing and finally dissolution of continuity. This condition is located most often at the level of the middle and lower thirds. Little, if any, callus forms and the factors of bone regeneration are largely lacking. The roentgenogram shows not only anterior angulation but considerable wasting of bone, with a tendency toward pointing of the fragments. The ends of the fragments become sclerotic. They may be held together by a small, tough band of fibrous tissue (Fig. 46).

Congenital pseudarthrosis has been treated successfully in many instances by the use of two or more massive bone grafts. Three tibial bone grafts, with additional amounts of osteoperiosteal bone, have been used successfully in the treatment of several cases which have come under our observation. The grafts must be sufficiently long to extend well above and well below

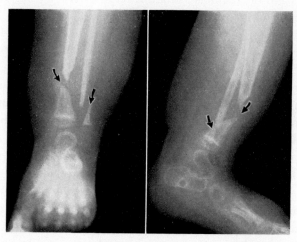

Fig. 46.—Infant, 18 months, with congenital pseudarthrosis of the tibia and fibula. The etiology of this condition is not clearly understood and routine bone graft procedures are usually unsuccessful.

the sclerosed and narrowed portion of the fragments of the tibia. *Attempts to obtain union by simply cutting off the ends of the fragments and bringing them together with wire or metal plates are ill conceived and doomed to failure.* After union has occurred, a long leg walking splint, with weight borne on the thigh or against the ischial tuberosity, should be used for a year or more. Re-fracture, caused by late absorption of bone as a result of invasion and replacement of grafts by hyperplastic fibrous tissue, has occurred frequently. Knowledge of this fact justifies a program of brace protection for 12 months or longer.

PART II

Fractures and Dislocations of

the Upper Extremity, Scapula and Clavicle

CHAPTER XVII

The Hand

No fractures and dislocations are more often neglected or so poorly treated as are those of the fingers and hand. From the standpoint of usefulness, the fingers, including the thumb, are the most important components of the upper extremity. Careless or indifferent treatment of sprained ligaments, small interphalangeal joint marginal fractures, avulsion of tendons or fractures of metacarpals or phalanges may lead to serious and permanent loss of function.

Every injured finger should be immobilized until torn structures have had time to repair, the fracture has healed, acute edema has subsided and extravasated blood has been absorbed. Immobilization should be restricted to the injured finger or fingers, *with the joints kept in flexion whenever possible.* Active exercise of the uninjured fingers is imperative, and it should be supervised by either the attending physician or his physical therapy assistant. The movement should be through a completely normal range and executed with strength and force. *Passive stretching should not be permitted; it merely produces additional injury, with edema and increased pain, and leads to greater stiffness and permanent disability.*

When the skin is broken in the region of an injury to a tendon or bone of the finger, emergency treatment must be instituted immediately if infection is to be prevented. Thorough cleansing with soap and water and operation under strict surgical precautions are essential. The wound should be carefully excised and thoroughly cleansed without using antiseptics. The skin edges should be drawn together loosely, burying little suture material within the wound. Lacerated tendons should be sutured before the skin is closed. If the injury is older than four hours, severed tendons should be loosely approximated to prevent retraction. If the wound heals by primary intention, secondary suture of the tendon may be carried out six weeks later. When suppuration occurs, four to six months or longer should elapse after healing of the wound before secondary tendon suture. Following suture of the wound, a large pressure dressing should be applied and the injured finger immediately splinted, with the *metacarpal joint and at least one of the interphalangeal joints in moderate flexion*.

We are in complete agreement with Bunnell, who has stressed the importance of the thumb. This digit should not be amputated even though all articulations are lost and only a rigid stump remains. The function of the hand will be infinitely better with a portion of the thumb than with no thumb. The stump will serve as a post or point of fixation against which objects may be held securely by the fingers.

INJURIES OF PHALANGES

FRACTURES OF THE PROXIMAL PHALANX.—Fractures of the phalanges most often occur in the proximal third of the proximal phalanx. The pull of the lumbrical and interosseous muscles, which normally flex the proximal and extend the distal phalanges, causes forward angulation at the site of the fracture (Fig. 47). Unless the fracture is oblique, with over-riding, it may be reduced by slight traction and forward flexion of the distal phalanges. *The finger should never be splinted in complete extension on a tongue depressor or any similar type of splint.* The

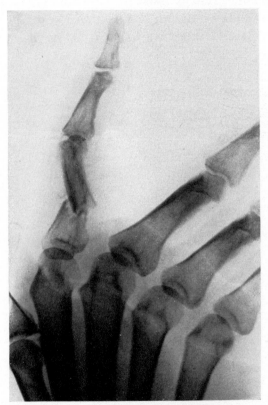

Fig. 47.—Fracture of proximal phalanx in poor position three weeks after injury.

proximal interphalangeal joint should be flexed almost as far as possible, while the metacarpal-phalangeal joint is flexed approximately 45 degrees (Fig. 48). A plaster cast applied to the forearm and the finger in which the fracture occurred, maintaining the position already described, will usually lead to union without deformity in four weeks and to a good functional result. Continuous traction may be applied with a small pin through the tough fibrous tissue of the distal end of the finger or through the bone of the phalanx distal to the fracture. Traction is obtained by rubber bands attached to a wire loop fastened to the cast at the wrist. The traction splint should be so arranged that

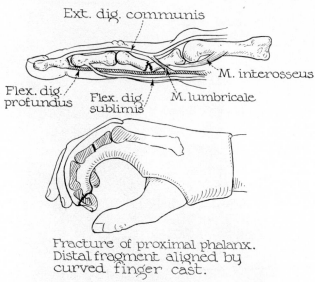

Ext. dig. communis

M. interosseus

Flex. dig.
profundus

Flex. dig.
sublimis

M. lumbricale

Fracture of proximal phalanx.
Distal fragment aligned by
curved finger cast.

Fig. 48.—Fracture of proximal phalanx with volar angulation. Only the involved finger is immobilized in plaster.

the tip of the flexed finger, regardless of which finger it may be, points toward the tubercle of the scaphoid bone of the wrist. In the normal hand the flexed fingers all converge toward this point.

FRACTURES OF THE MIDDLE PHALANX.—Fractures across the middle phalanx may lead to forward or backward angulation of the bone, depending on which side of the insertion of the flexor sublimis tendon the break occurs (Fig. 49). If the fracture is distal to its attachment to the phalanx, the proximal fragment will be flexed, with volar angulation of the finger, and reduction is accomplished by flexion of the digit. When the fracture is proximal, the distal fragment is flexed and reduction is achieved by extension. The fracture is immobilized as illustrated.

FRACTURES OF THE DISTAL PHALANX.—Crushing injuries and

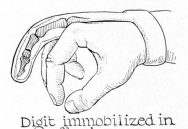

Fracture of middle phalanx proximal to insertion of flexor dig. sublimis tendon. Aligned by extension

Fracture of middle phalanx distal to insertion of flexor dig. sublimis tendon. Reduce by flexion

Digit immobilized in flexion

FIG. 49.—Use of a tongue blade as the splint for these fractures is ill advised. The metacarpal-phalangeal joint should *never* be immobilized in extension. Simple plaster dressing for the fractured finger insures a good functional result.

hence comminuted fractures are most common in the distal phalanx. Displacement of the fragments is rare. Treatment consists of protection of the end of the finger for 10 to 14 days by a wooden or metal splint. If the soft structures of the finger-tip are lost, with exposure of the end of the phalanx, a primary full thickness skin graft should be applied. In all such instances, every effort should be made to salvage the end of the finger.

SPRAINS, SUBLUXATIONS OR DISLOCATIONS OF FINGER JOINTS. These differ principally in degree. They are produced by the same type of injury. Forced backward displacement of a finger may cause a sprain of the anterior capsule of one or more of the interphalangeal joints, a dislocation of an interphalangeal joint or a fracture-dislocation in which there are chip fractures from the joint margin. Reduction of the dislocation or fracture-dislocation is readily performed by applying traction and flexing the finger. A very light plaster of paris dressing, applied directly to the skin, with the finger held in moderate interphalangeal joint flexion for two to three weeks, is the treatment of choice. Stiffness in the injured joint is the common finding after the splint is removed. No forced motion or stretching should be permitted. Active use of the hand will bring about a gradual but much more certain recovery of function. Six to eight months may elapse before full recovery is attained. Paraffin baths are the most useful form of physical therapy.

PARAFFIN BATHS

Place five packages of ordinary paraffin used in sealing fruit jars and 1 pt. of mineral oil in a deep oval dishpan large enough to accommodate the entire hand with fingers extended. Heat over a flame until the paraffin has melted and has mixed with the mineral oil. Turn off the flame. Allow the paraffin to cool until a scum forms on the surface. Quickly run the hand through the paraffin, and allow the coating to set. Do not flex or extend the fingers; motion will crack the paraffin. Repeat five times. Each time allow the paraffin to harden. Now remove the accumulated paraffin from the hand and set it aside on a piece of clean paper. Repeat this procedure four or five times so that the hand is placed in the melted paraffin 25 or 30 times. At the end of the treatment, all of the paraffin is replaced in the pan, which is covered and set aside until the next treatment. Paraffin baths are most effective when used twice each day.

INJURIES OF THE FIRST METACARPAL
(THUMB) BONE

FRACTURES OF THE SHAFT.—These fractures, with the exception of the Bennett fracture and dislocation of the proximally placed epiphysis, differ little from those affecting the other metacarpal bones. The fracture line may be oblique, spiral or transverse, with or without angulation or over-riding. Comminuted and open fractures are encountered frequently because of the exposed position of the thumb. If the fragments can be accurately aligned and the reduction is stable, a plaster cast extending from the proximal part of the forearm onto the abducted and opposed thumb will maintain the position and permit continued use of the uninvolved fingers. Unstable or badly comminuted fractures require continuous traction as used for the Bennett fracture (Fig. 50). Fractures of the shaft should be immobilized for a period of six weeks.

BENNETT FRACTURE.—This is in reality a fracture-dislocation. It results from a blow directed upward through the longitudinal axis of the thumb or from a fall on the abducted digit. The oblique fracture line extends from the medial aspect of the proximal end of the shaft upward and laterally into the metacarpal-multangular joint. The small medial fragment remains in situ while the main lateral portion of the metacarpal bone and attached phalanges are dislocated dorsally and proximally. Since the usefulness of the thumb is dependent on its wide range of painless motion at the carpal-metacarpal joint, the Bennett fracture must be accurately reduced and maintained until solid union has occurred (Fig. 50).

Reduction is not difficult to obtain by skeletal traction. The position cannot be maintained by an ordinary plaster dressing because of the obliquity of the fracture and because the metacarpal slides proximally on the saddle-shaped surface of the multangular major bone. The plaster cast must be molded to the lateral side of the base of the thumb to help stabilize the fracture and close the gap between the fragments. After six weeks, union should be strong enough to permit guarded use of the thumb. Inadequate reduction will result in instability and

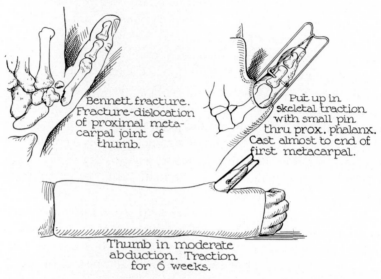

Bennett fracture.
Fracture-dislocation
of proximal meta-
carpal joint of
thumb.

Put up in
skeletal traction
with small pin
thru prox. phalanx.
Cast almost to end of
first metacarpal.

Thumb in moderate
abduction. Traction
for 6 weeks.

FIG. 50.—Skeletal traction is required for reduction of the Bennett fracture—dislocation of the metacarpal-carpal joint of the thumb. Inadequate reposition of fragments results in arthritis, pain and loss of function. The web between thumb and index finger must be adequately padded to prevent pressure sores.

pain from secondary degenerative changes in the metacarpal-carpal articulation.

DISLOCATION OF THE METACARPAL-PHALANGEAL JOINT.— A hard blow on the hyperextended thumb may result in a posterior dislocation of the proximal phalanx as the head of the metacarpal bone is forced through a rent in the anterior capsule of the metacarpal-phalangeal joint (Fig. 51). In most cases, reduction can be accomplished by traction on the markedly abducted thumb while pressure is exerted against the base of the proximal phalanx. As the phalanx is felt to engage the meta-carpal head, the reduction is completed by flexion of the thumb,

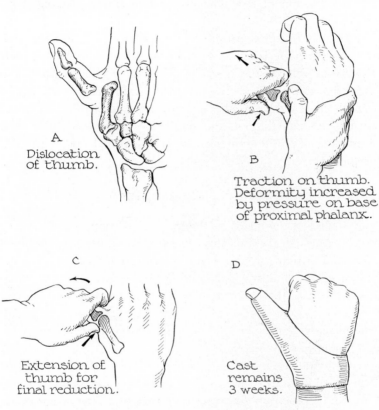

A
Dislocation
of thumb.

B

Traction on thumb.
Deformity increased
by pressure on base
of proximal phalanx.

C

D

Extension of
thumb for
final reduction.

Cast
remains
3 weeks.

Fig. 51.—Treatment of dislocation of the thumb.

which is then immobilized in a neutral position for three weeks by a plaster dressing extending from the forearm to the distal phalanx.

Not infrequently the small tear in the capsule is so constricted just above the large head of the metacarpal bone that reduction can be obtained only by surgical means. Through a lateral incision, tendons which may be caught between the bones are retracted while the hole in the capsule is enlarged sufficiently to allow retraction of the metacarpal bone and reposition of the phalanx.

Rarely is the phalanx dislocated anteriorly. When this does occur, reduction is obtained by hyperflexion of the thumb. Epiphyseal separations at the base of the first metacarpal bone are reduced by manual traction while firm pressure is applied over the base of the distal fragment. Since epiphyseal separation occurs only in children, the possibility of growth arrest with shortening of the thumb must be kept in mind and a guarded prognosis given.

Injuries of Second to Fifth Metacarpal Bones

Fractures of the metacarpal bones result from a blow directed upward through the knuckles or against the dorsum of the hand or from a crushing injury. The history of such an injury and the presence of pain, swelling, crepitus, prominence of the metacarpal head in the palm or shortening of the shaft as indicated by mal-alignment of the knuckles suggest a metacarpal fracture. The displacement or angulation is influenced more by the fracture force than by muscle pull.

Transverse Fractures of the Shaft.—*With posterior angulation* such fractures are treated by correction of alignment and fixation for six weeks by means of a plaster cast dressing applied to the back of the forearm, hand and finger, with the metacarpal-phalangeal joint flexed. Proximal and dorsal displacement of the lower fragment may be corrected by posterior angulation and extension of the distal fragment after engaging the ends of the bone (Fig. 52). If reduction cannot be accomplished by this method, skeletal traction is indicated. Open reduction is rarely necessary.

MULTIPLE FRACTURES of metacarpal bones with gross displacement of the fragments usually require skeletal traction to each digit. A forearm cast is applied incorporating a curved volar metal splint for each involved finger. Traction is applied to each finger *with all joints in flexion* as for a single metacarpal

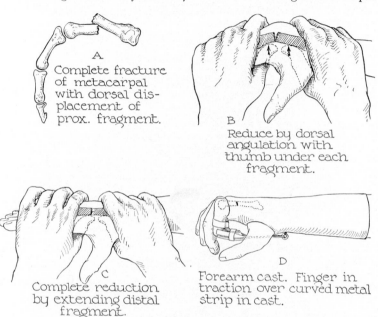

A
Complete fracture
of metacarpal
with dorsal dis-
placement of
prox. fragment.

B
Reduce by dorsal
angulation with
thumb under each
fragment.

C
Complete reduction
by extending distal
fragment.

D
Forearm cast. Finger in
traction over curved metal
strip in cast.

FIG. 52.—Method of reduction and recommended type of immobilization for transverse fracture of a metacarpal bone.

fracture. If open reduction is necessary, continuous traction may be required to maintain position and alignment; or internal fixation may be achieved by threaded wires which traverse the fragments and engage the adjacent metacarpal bones. The wires are cut off beneath the skin and removed after healing is complete.

OBLIQUE OR SPIRAL FRACTURES without displacement are immobilized for six weeks. When the lower fragment is displaced sufficiently to cause shortening, skeletal traction for four to six weeks, as described for the Bennett fracture, is the method of choice (Fig. 53).

FRACTURES OF THE NECK.—Such fractures, with forward displacement of the distal end into the palm of the hand, are common. For restoration of normal function, the alignment must

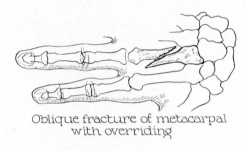

Oblique fracture of metacarpal
with overriding

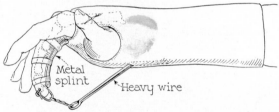

Metal
splint   Heavy wire

Traction by skeletal traction-pin through
distal phalanx. Finger joints flexed over metal
in cast from just behind knuckle to upper ⅓ arm.

FIG. 53.—Accurate reduction and immobilization of oblique or comminuted fractures of a metacarpal bone requires skeletal traction. Note flexion of finger joints.

be accurately restored. Reduction is accomplished by upward pressure on the metacarpal head through the flexed metacarpal-phalangeal joint while pushing downward on the distal end of the upper fragment (Fig. 54). It is not possible to reduce this fracture by traction on the extended finger, since the capsule and ligaments of the metacarpal-phalangeal joint are taut only in flexion. A plaster of paris dressing affords secure fixation. In unstable fractures the cast should be applied in two stages. The first section of the cast should extend from the forearm to the fracture site. After this plaster has hardened, the dressing is continued onto the flexed finger, while upward pressure on the metacarpal head is maintained. Union sufficient to allow guarded use of the finger is usually adequate within four weeks.

Post-Reduction Care.—Plaster dressings for metacarpal fractures should be as simple as possible. Free use of the uninjured

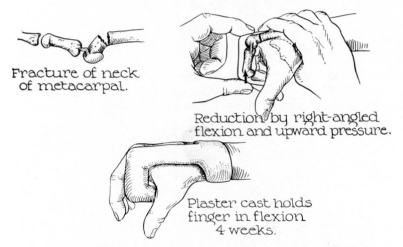

Fracture of neck
of metacarpal.

Reduction by right-angled
flexion and upward pressure.

Plaster cast holds
finger in flexion
4 weeks.

Fig. 54.—This closed fracture is too often badly managed. Malunion leaves the hand crippled because of inability to grasp firmly due to displacement of the head of the metacarpal bone into the palm.

fingers must be encouraged to prevent prolonged convalescence and permanent disability of the hand as a result of stiffness due to capsular contraction or the formation of dense adhesions.

DISLOCATIONS OF METACARPAL-PHALANGEAL JOINTS.—Dislocations occur most frequently in the posterior direction, although, rarely, the phalanx may be displaced anteriorly or to either side. If reduction is not successful by manual traction on the extended finger, the digit should be hyperextended while the proximal phalanx is pushed over the metacarpal head by firm pressure at its base, followed by flexion of the finger. Occasionally, surgical intervention is necessary in order to enlarge the opening in the capsule of the joint. A plaster of paris dressing is the safe method of immobilization. *Only the involved finger is immobilized.* A position of flexion should be maintained for three weeks.

AVULSION OF EXTENSOR TENDON OF FINGER

This lesion, the baseball or mallet finger, is produced by a blow to the tip of the finger which forces the distal phalanx into

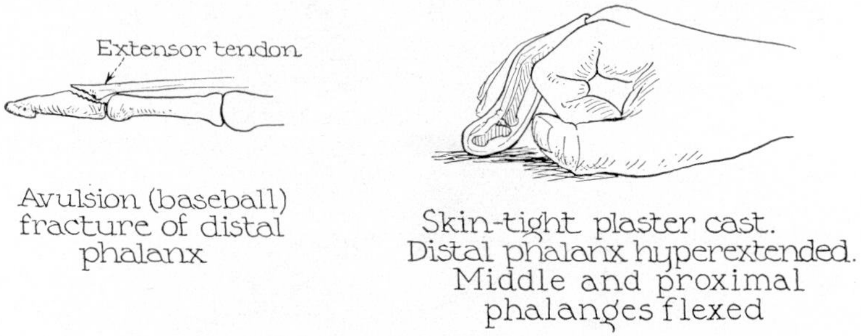

Extensor tendon

Avulsion (baseball) fracture of distal phalanx

Skin-tight plaster cast. Distal phalanx hyperextended. Middle and proximal phalanges flexed

FIG. 55.—Closed treatment of mallet finger.

flexion. Injuries of this type may occur when catching a baseball or when tucking the sheet under a mattress. The loss of ability to extend the distal phalanx actively while passive motion remains normal is indicative of an avulsion of the extensor tendon from its insertion onto the proximal dorsal margin of the distal phalanx. The forced flexion of the end of the finger against the contracting extensor muscle may simultaneously tear off a small fragment of bone to which the tendon is attached. In such cases, the history and physical findings may be supplemented by definite roentgen evidence.

A plaster cast dressing should maintain hyperextension of the distal phalanx *while the proximal interphalangeal and the meta-carpal-phalangeal joints are flexed* for six weeks. If the position is maintained sufficiently long there usually will be complete recovery of function (Fig. 55). Surgical intervention is not only technically difficult but rarely necessary even in old cases, and all patients should be given the benefit of adequate conservative care before operative repair is advised. The results of open reduction have been disappointing.

CHAPTER XVIII

The Wrist

THIS chapter is limited to the discussion of injuries to the carpal bones and dislocations involving the radial-carpal joint. Colles' fracture and epiphyseal injuries involving the bones of the forearm at the wrist are described in Chapter XIX.

SPRAIN OF THE WRIST

An injury to the hand which is followed by swelling of the wrist and pain on movement of the wrist, with no roentgenographic evidence of fracture or dislocation, should be recognized as a sprain. The symptoms are most effectively relieved by a light anterior plaster splint or a circular cast. After 21 days the splint should be removed and additional roentgen studies, including oblique views, made. If there is still no evidence of a fracture of the navicular bone, the cast may be discarded and active movements of the fingers and wrist encouraged. These exercises are more easily performed with the hand and wrist submerged in a warm water bath. *Recovery will be prolonged rather than shortened by forced movement or vigorous massage.*

DISLOCATION OF THE LUNATE BONE

An interesting and not uncommon injury which may result from a fall on the outstretched and hyperextended hand is a

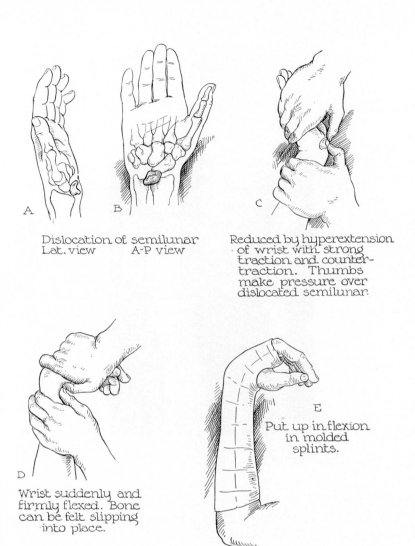

Dislocation of semilunar
Lat. view   A-P view

Reduced by hyperextension
of wrist with strong
traction and counter-
traction. Thumbs
make pressure over
dislocated semilunar.

Wrist suddenly and
firmly flexed. Bone
can be felt slipping
into place.

E
Put up in flexion
in molded
splints.

Fig. 56.—Manipulative reduction of dislocation of lunate bone of the wrist.

143

forward dislocation of the lunate or semilunar bone. As the posterior ligaments between the lunate and capitate distally and the
radius proximally are ruptured, the lunate rotates *anteriorly* and
comes to lie beneath the flexor tendons and the volar carpal
ligament. The patient will then hold the wrist in a position of

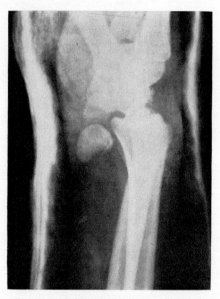

Fig. 57.—Lateral roentgenogram showing anterior dislocation of lunate
bone and proximal half of the navicular.

flexion in order to release the tension over the displaced bone,
which can be palpated on deep digital pressure.

ROENTGENOGRAMS will show the capitate bone in contact
with the articular surface of the radius and the lunate in abnor-
mal position in front of the wrist (Figs. 56 and 57).

REDUCTION by the Conwell method can be accomplished
under local anesthesia or Pentothal sodium.

TECHNIQUE OF REDUCTION

1. Forcefully distract the wrist, to displace the capitate distally and to open up a space for the lunate. (One assistant should pull down on the hand while a second assistant pulls up on the flexed elbow.)

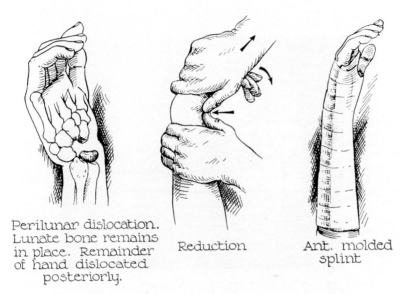

Perilunar dislocation. Lunate bone remains in place. Remainder of hand dislocated posteriorly.

Reduction

Ant. molded splint

Fig. 58.—Reduction of perilunar dislocation of the wrist.

2. While maintaining distraction, hyperextend the wrist.
3. The operator's thumbs must mold the lunate distally and backward as the wrist is suddenly brought from acute extension to acute flexion. If reduction is accomplished there will be felt or heard a sudden snap, and full motion of the wrist will be possible immediately.

Boehler states that continuous longitudinal traction on the extended fingers for 10 minutes, timed by a clock, with countertraction on the elbow flexed to a right angle, will invariably lead to reduction of the lunate by forces brought to play against it by the taut flexor tendons.

IMMOBILIZATION should be maintained for three weeks in slight flexion by anterior and posterior plaster splints *which should not interfere with movement of the fingers.* The total period of disability usually ranges from six to eight weeks.

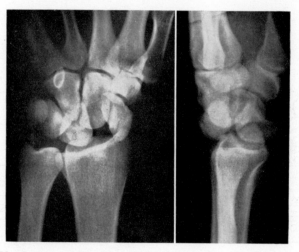

FIG. 59.—Perilunar dislocation of wrist. Note loss of normal relationship of carpal bones in anteroposterior view and dorsal dislocation of the carpus around the undisturbed lunate shown in the lateral view.

Less commonly, the lunate may be *dislocated posteriorly.* Reduction is accomplished as for anterior dislocation with the exception that the wrist must be acutely extended from a flexed position in order to complete the manipulation and then immobilized in slight extension.

There may be an associated fracture of the carpal navicular, and its proximal fragment may be dislocated with the lunate. Following reduction, immobilization in a forearm cast which includes the thumb must be continued until there is roentgen evidence of union. This may require as long as six months.

Backward dislocation of the hand and carpal bones, leaving the lunate bone in position, is exceedingly rare but may occur. This is known as a *perilunar dislocation* (Figs. 58 and 59).

Unreduced dislocations of the lunate cannot be treated successfully by manipulation after three weeks from the time of injury, and there is a difference of opinion as to whether open

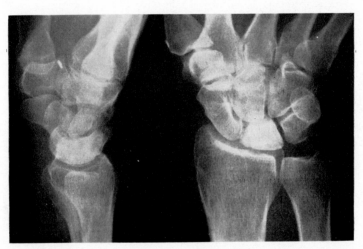

Fig. 60.—Aseptic necrosis of lunate bone (Kienböck's disease) may be mistaken for fracture when fragmentation of the devitalized bone occurs while it is undergoing replacement by creeping substitution.

reduction or excision of the bone is the better method of treatment. Watson-Jones reports that of 12 patients on whom he performed open reductions, 11 had painful wrists due to *aseptic necrosis* of the lunate bone and degenerative arthritis in the surrounding joints; this indicates that excision of the bone is the method of choice. Aseptic necrosis of the lunate bone, which occasionally occurs without a fracture or dislocation, is known as *Kienböck's disease* (Fig. 60). Note the high density of the lunate compared to the atrophic surrounding living bone.

FRACTURES OF THE NAVICULAR BONE

The carpal scaphoid or navicular bone, together with the lunate, is interposed between the hand and the distal end of the radius. The bean-shaped navicular bone is divided by a constricted region called the waist into an extra-articular distal

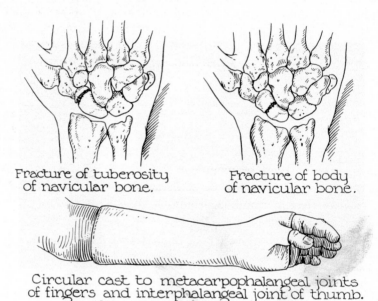

Fracture of tuberosity
of navicular bone.

Fracture of body
of navicular bone.

Circular cast to metacarpophalangeal joints
of fingers and interphalangeal joint of thumb.
Hand in very slight dorsiflexion.

Fig. 61.—Treatment of recent fracture of the carpal navicular (scaphoid) bone.

portion, or tubercle, and a larger proximal intra-articular segment, or body. Forces transmitted through the hand to the radius may fracture the navicular bone, particularly if the carpus is in a position of slight dorsiflexion and radial deviation. The fracture line may cross the tubercle, the waist or the body of the bone.

The patient with a navicular fracture complains of severe

local pain and loss of wrist motion, particularly on abduction
and extension. Physical examination reveals swelling and tenderness in the anatomic snuffbox and over the dorsum of the wrist.
After every severe injury to the wrist roentgenograms should be
made in multiple planes. Because of the forward tilt of the bone,
some fractures are demonstrable only in oblique views. For the
same reason, slight dorsiflexion of the wrist is the best position
for obtaining a sharply profiled anteroposterior view.

TREATMENT.—The wrist should be immobilized with the hand
in slight dorsiflexion and radial deviation (Fig. 61). The circular
plaster dressing applied over stockinette without padding extends
from the forearm to the metacarpal-phalangeal joints of the second to fifth fingers and to the interphalangeal joint of the thumb,
with the latter in a position of opposition. Although union is
usually complete in eight to 12 weeks, continuous and adequate
immobilization must be maintained until there is unmistakable
roentgenographic evidence of obliteration of the fracture line.
This may require continued splinting for six months or even
longer.

Hair line or fissure fractures of the navicular bone are difficult
to demonstrate and are frequently overlooked on the first roentgen films. An acutely sprained wrist should be immobilized in
plaster, even when the roentgenograms appear negative for a
fracture. After three to four weeks, the roentgen examination
should be repeated. A previously concealed fissure fracture may
now be demonstrated, due to decalcification and absorption
along the margins of the fracture. This important feature of
navicular fractures cannot be overemphasized.

Nonunion.—The failure of union of fractures of the navicular
bone may be attributed to failure to recognize a fissure fracture,
inadequate and insufficiently prolonged immobilization, or to
death of one fragment resulting from aseptic necrosis. Because
of the arrangement of blood vessels entering the bone, the proximal fragment is most frequently deprived of its nutrition by the

Two nutrient arteries. Fracture does not result in necrosis of either fragment.

One nutrient artery. Necrosis results when fracture disrupts arterial supply of fragment.

One nutrient artery centrally placed. Necrosis occurs in fragment excluded from blood supply.

Fig. 62.—Blood supply of the carpal navicular bone. Fracture may cause necrosis of avascular fragments.

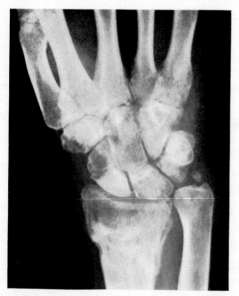

Fig. 63.—Union of fracture of navicular bone although the proximal fragment is necrotic from interruption of its blood supply. The patient will be rewarded with a good functional result if the wrist is protected from performing strenuous work during the period required for replacement of the dead bone by living bone.

fracture (Fig. 62). The tubercle is adequately supplied with vessels, so fractures here heal within six weeks, and rarely, if ever, is necrosis observed. Avascular necrosis of one fragment jeopardizes the chances of union, and although consolidation may occur, late arthritic changes in the wrist are common (Fig. 63). The dead fragment cannot be recognized on roentgenograms immediately following the injury but is evident after a

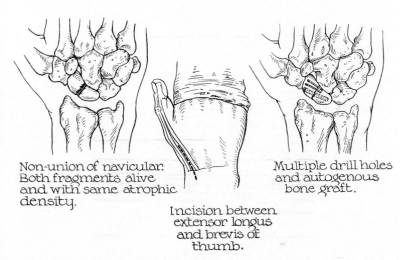

Non-union of navicular.
Both fragments alive
and with same atrophic
density.

Incision between
extensor longus
and brevis of
thumb.

Multiple drill holes
and autogenous
bone graft.

Fig. 64.—Treatment of nonunion of fracture of the navicular (scaphoid) bone of the wrist.

period of immobilization in a cast. The distal living fragment of bone will undergo atrophy from disuse of the wrist, while the proximal dead portion, without blood supply, will retain its original density. The resulting contrast in density on the roentgenogram is the earliest sign of this vascular complication. As new blood vessels grow into and cause replacement of the dead fragment by the process of creeping substitution, late roentgenograms will show a progressive, irregular appearance of the bone, with thinning of the cartilage space between the navicular and the distal end of the radius.

TREATMENT.—Established nonunion with two live fragments, associated with pain in the wrist, is best treated by multiple drilling and the insertion of a bone graft. The radial aspect of the bone is exposed through an incision in the anatomic snuff-box. One cortical bone graft from the excised radial styloid process or proximal third of the ulna should be inserted into as

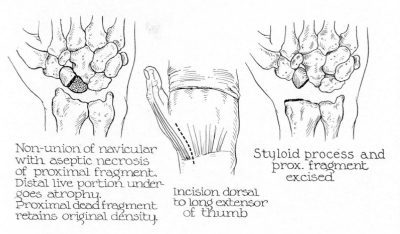

Non-union of navicular with aseptic necrosis of proximal fragment. Distal live portion undergoes atrophy. Proximal dead fragment retains original density.

Incision dorsal to long extensor of thumb

Styloid process and prox. fragment excised

FIG. 65.—Treatment of aseptic necrosis of the navicular bone of the wrist.

large a channel as possible to extend from the distal into the proximal fragment (Fig. 64). Care must be exercised to prevent damage to the articular cartilage by the drill or the graft. The wrist should be immobilized as for a recent fracture until union is established by roentgenographic examinations. It is wise to protect the wrist by means of a removable molded leather metal-reinforced, cock-up splint for an additional three months. This will permit the patient to exercise the wrist while final consolidation occurs. A firm fibrous union may result in a painless and serviceable wrist, but the goal of treatment should be bony union of the fragments.

A painful wrist resulting from an established *nonunion with a dead proximal fragment* is best treated by surgical removal of the devitalized portion *and the styloid process of the radius* (Fig. 65). When the dead fragment has been unrecognized for several years and there is pain in the wrist due to secondary arthritis involving the proximal row of carpal bones, an arthrodesis of the carpus to the radius, utilizing a tibial bone graft, is the treatment of choice.

CHAPTER XIX

The Forearm

FRACTURES OF THE DISTAL END OF THE RADIUS

FRACTURES of the distal end of the radius include the following types: hyperextension (Colles'); flexion (reversed Colles' or Smith's); posterior marginal (Barton's); anterior marginal (reversed Barton's), and fracture-dislocation of the distal radial epiphysis (Fig. 66).

The most common bone injury occurring in the region of the wrist is a Colles' fracture, which results from an attempt to arrest a fall by the outstretched arm and hand. This same trauma in very young children produces a greenstick fracture several inches above the lower extremity of the radius or ulna or a supracondylar fracture of the humerus. In youngsters over the age of 10 and in adolescents, a fracture-dislocation of the distal radial epiphysis is not uncommon.

Accurate reduction of fractures around the wrist joint must include restoration of the normal relationships of the bones which enter into this complex articulation and on which wrist function depends. Any surgeon who undertakes the treatment of injuries to the bones and joints should *be familiar with these important anatomic relationships*. The following are things to remember about the wrist:

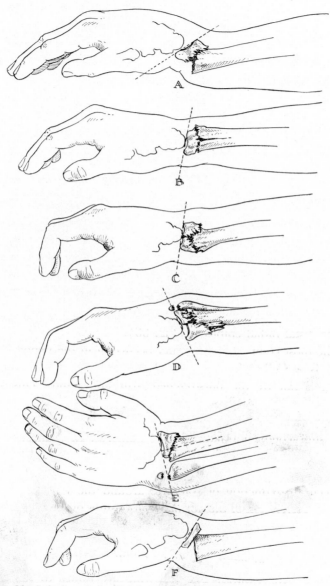

FIG. 66.—Injuries of the distal end of the radius which may disturb the articular plane and impair function of the wrist joint.

1. The radius is normally ½ in. longer than the ulna.

2. In the anteroposterior view, the articular surface of the radius slopes from its styloid process proximally toward the ulna, creating an angle of about 25 degrees.

3. In the lateral view, the plane of the articular surface faces forward and volarward at an angle of approximately 15 degrees. This is called the angle of articulation and is most important to the function of the wrist joint (Fig. 67).

Colles' Fractures

DIAGNOSIS.—Colles' fracture is definitely suggested by the history of a fall on the outstretched hand with resulting pain and loss of function of the wrist and the finding of tenderness over the end of the radius, with swelling, shortening of the radius and broadening of the wrist. This common fracture was first described in 1814 by Abraham Colles, an Irish surgeon. It presents the following anatomic characteristics:

1. A fracture of the distal end of the radius within 1 in. of the wrist joint, and frequently also a fracture of the ulnar styloid.

2. Involvement of the whole thickness of the distal shaft of the radius, with possible fragmentation of its articular surface.

3. Backward displacement of the distal radial fragment with or without impaction into the lower end of the proximal fragment.

4. Radial displacement of the distal fragment.

5. Changes in position of the fracture fragments producing a reverse of the articular angles and the characteristic silver fork deformity.

    a) The articular surface of the distal end of the radius now faces down and back instead of down and forward.

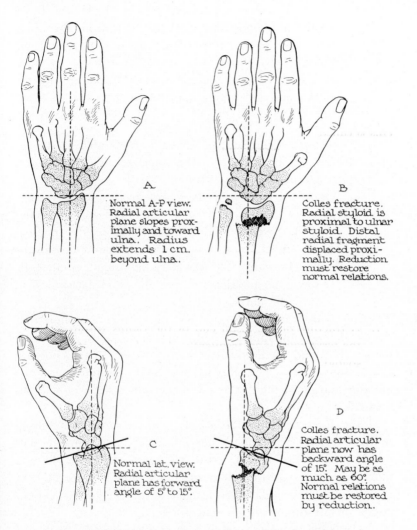

A

Normal A-P view.
Radial articular
plane slopes prox-
imally and toward
ulna. Radius
extends 1 cm.
beyond ulna.

B

Colles fracture.
Radial styloid is
proximal to ulnar
styloid. Distal
radial fragment
displaced proxi-
mally. Reduction
must restore
normal relations.

C

Normal lat. view.
Radial articular
plane has forward
angle of 5° to 15°.

D

Colles fracture.
Radial articular
plane now has
backward angle
of 15°. May be as
much as 60°.
Normal relations
must be restored
by reduction.

Fig. 67.—Anatomic relations of the radius at the wrist and how they are disarranged by Colles' fracture.

157

b) In the anteroposterior view the slope from the tip of the styloid process toward the ulna may be completely reversed.

c) If there is impaction or marked displacement, the radius may be shorter than the ulna.

TREATMENT

1. *Reduction.*—Pentothal anesthesia is preferable in the reduction of Colles' fracture, but local procaine anesthesia is quite acceptable (Fig. 68).

   a) Grasp the hand as in the act of shaking hands.

   b) Break up the impaction, if present. Force the hand backward while exerting traction and countertraction.

   c) Apply direct traction and force the hand downward and ulnarward. The distal radial fragment must be restored to position by pushing it volarward and toward the ulna.

The reduction should be perfect. Examination should show that the distal end of the radial styloid is now from $\frac{1}{4}$ to $\frac{1}{2}$ in. distal to the distal end of the ulnar styloid. A lateral roentgenogram should show that a line drawn between the posterior and the anterior margin of the distal end of the radius slopes down and forward.

If the fracture is not accurately reduced and immobilized until after solid bony union has taken place, healing in malposition may cause a weak wrist, pain, gross deformity, limited movement, tenosynovitis, ulnar instability and pain because of rupture of the triangular fibrocartilage of the ulnar-radial articulation, or late rupture of the extensor tendons.

2. *Immobilization.*—Note that short fiber board, cardboard or metal splints are altogether inadequate for safe immobilization of any fracture of the bones of the forearm.

   A. If there is *no fragmentation* of the distal segment and if the reduction is accurate, the splinting does not

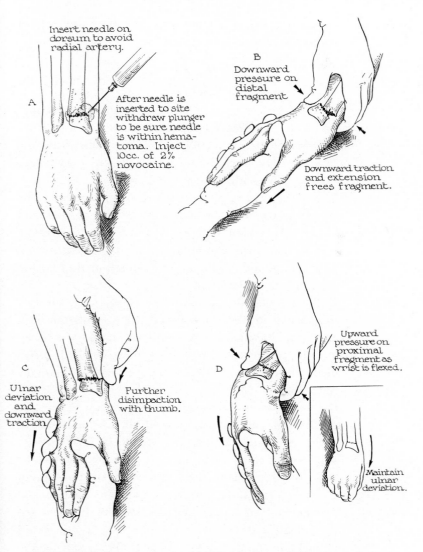

Fig. 68.—Technique of reduction of Colles' fracture with local anesthesia.

159

necessarily have to extend above the elbow, but it must include the hand to (though not across) the meta-carpal-phalangeal joints.

(1) The ideal method of immobilization is by means of anterior and posterior plaster slabs with little padding (Fig. 69). (Excessive padding may permit loss of position of the fragments.)

(2) While the reduction is being maintained, the slabs are carefully molded to the arm and bound together with a gauze bandage.

(3) The surgeon should use good judgment. The bandage must be sufficiently secure to maintain the reduction but not tight enough to interfere with the circulation.

(4) The position of the hand should be that of flexion and ulnar deviation.

B. If the *fracture of the radius is comminuted,* the cast should extend above the flexed elbow, with the fore-arm in midposition between supination and pronation, in order to prevent rotary strain and possible displacement of fragments. This is the position of anatomic rest.

C. If *comminution is extreme* and includes more than the distal 1 in. of the radius, or if the carpus tends to subluxate, continuous traction should be used.

(1) A Kirschner wire or threaded pin should be passed through the midportion of the thumb metacarpal. This provides adequate traction and at the same time deviates the hand ulnarward (Fig. 71).

(2) While traction is maintained, after reducing the fracture, a plaster cast should be applied, incorporating the pin. To be effective this cast must extend above the elbow. *The fingers and thumb*

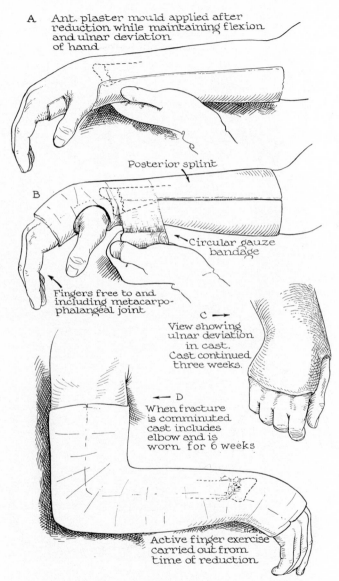

A Ant. plaster mould applied after reduction while maintaining flexion and ulnar deviation of hand

Posterior splint

B

Circular gauze bandage

Fingers free to and including metacarpo-phalangeal joint

C →
View showing ulnar deviation in cast. Cast continued three weeks.

← D
When fracture is comminuted cast includes elbow and is worn for 6 weeks

Active finger exercise carried out from time of reduction

Fig. 69.—Application of anterior and posterior plaster molds.

161

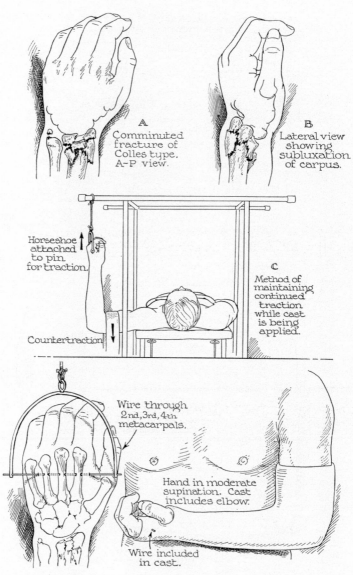

A

Comminuted fracture of Colles type. A-P view.

B

Lateral view showing subluxation of carpus.

Horseshoe attached to pin for traction.

C

Method of maintaining continued traction while cast is being applied.

Countertraction

Wire through 2nd, 3rd, 4th metacarpals.

Hand in moderate supination. Cast includes elbow.

Wire included in cast.

FIG. 70.—Skeletal traction for reduction and immobilization of severely comminuted fractures of the distal end of the radius.

162

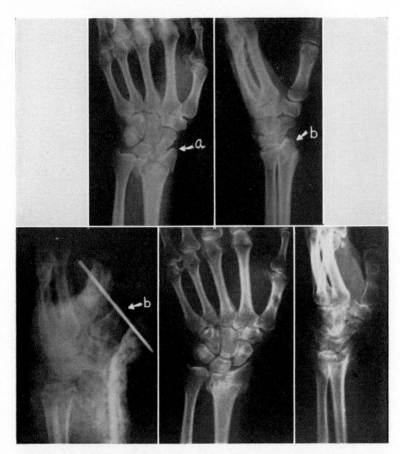

Fig. 71.—Severely comminuted Colles' fracture of the distal end of the radius, with posterior displacement, *a*. Treated by traction with a pin through the first metacarpal, *b*. The pin is incorporated into a plaster cast while traction is being maintained. Use of skeletal traction has greatly improved the anatomic and functional end-result for this injury.

163

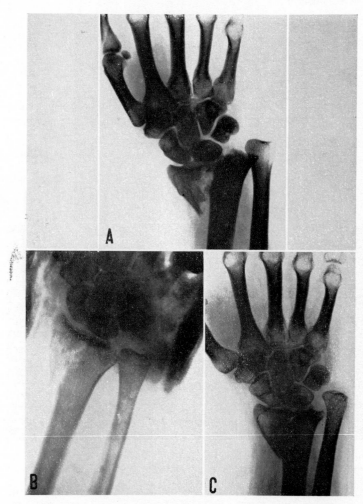

Fig. 72.—Disastrous result of discontinuing immobilization too soon in comminuted fracture of the radius with dislocation of the wrist (*A*). Satisfactory reduction was obtained by skeletal traction with a threaded pin passed through three metacarpal bones and then incorporated in a plaster cast (*B*). When the pin was removed after 3½ weeks, position was lost and fracture healed with shortening of radius and deformity (*C*). Immobilization should have been continued at least two weeks longer.

*should be exercised vigorously and frequently
each day.* A forearm cast will suffice if a second
pin is placed through the proximal third of the
ulna.

(3) The metal pin or pins may be removed after four
weeks, but immobilization should be continued
for two to three weeks longer (Fig. 72).

(4) Open operations should not be necessary in dealing with fractures of the distal end of the radius
or ulna.

POSTREDUCTION CARE.—1. Immediately after the application
of the plaster dressing, anteroposterior and lateral roentgenograms should be made to ascertain the accuracy of the reduction.
These should be taken in the operating room and the reduction
adjusted if necessary before the patient is allowed to awaken
from a general anesthetic.

2. If the articular surface of the radius has not been restored
to its normal relationships or if the radial deviation of the distal
fragment has not been corrected, the cast should be removed
and further attempts at reduction made until roentgenograms
show that the reduction is accurate.

3. The patient is warned to keep the part elevated and he
should be seen within 24 hours of the reduction to make sure
that swelling of the arm within the cast is not restricting the
circulation of the hand.

4. If there is excessive swelling or ischemia, the plaster
dressing must be loosened at once. Even temporary loss of the
reduction must be permitted if necessary to prevent Volkmann's
contracture or ischemic necrosis.

5. As swelling subsides, the slack in the dressing may be
eliminated by binding the plaster splints more tightly together
with a woven elastic bandage.

6. *It is imperative* to get roentgenograms after seven to 10
days in all instances to determine that the reduction has not

been lost. Failure to do so is considered negligence in the eyes of the court and may be the only means whereby the physician can be prosecuted for an unfavorable result.

7. The arm should *not be carried* in a sling for more than two to three days.

8. A satisfactory functional result requires that the patient be instructed over and over again in the active use of the fingers. He should be encouraged to use the hand as freely as possible throughout the period of healing of the fracture.

9. The arm must be moved through a complete range of shoulder joint motion several times each day if the complication of "frozen shoulder" is to be avoided. When the shoulder is not exercised and the arm is maintained at the side, muscles and tendons may become adherent to their sheaths and adhesions may form in the shoulder joint capsule, causing pain and restriction of motion. This rarely happens in children, but is common in older or elderly patients. Pain and restricted shoulder movements, caused by irritation at the insertion of the supraspinatus tendon, are common and are ordinarily relieved by the injection of procaine into the tender spot.

10. The trauma which produces fracture of the wrist may also cause bruising and contusions of muscles and bursae at the shoulder. If shoulder exercises are not insisted on, edema and adhesions may involve trunks of the brachial plexus. There may follow vasomotor disturbances consisting of swelling of the hand, wrist and forearm, intractable pain and trophic changes in the skin of the hand and forearm. These constitute a most unhappy symptom complex, not fully understood and slow to respond to treatment, which has been designated *causalgia*.

11. Simple Colles' fractures should be immobilized for three weeks. The wrist should be brought from the position of acute flexion to neutral in two weeks.

12. Continuous immobilization for five to seven weeks is indicated when there is fragmentation of the distal fragment.

13. Function returns slowly after removal of the cast. An accurate reduction does not assure the patient full active motion, and frequently excellent function is obtained even though the deformity has not been corrected.

MALUNITED COLLES' FRACTURE.—If the union has not completely consolidated, the patient should be anesthetized with Pentothal sodium, ether or gas, and the impaction and early

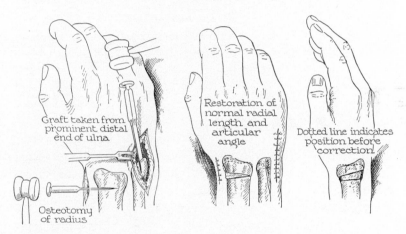

Graft taken from prominent distal end of ulna

Osteotomy of radius

Restoration of normal radial length and articular angle

Dotted line indicates position before correction

FIG. 73.—Campbell-Burrows operation for correction of malunion of Colles' fracture.

union should be broken up with forceful manual manipulation or with a Thomas wrench. The fracture may then be reduced and the arm immobilized for four to six weeks.

Bony union of mal-aligned Colles' fractures with pain and poor function may be corrected by open operation. We prefer the Campbell-Burrows operation (Fig. 73). An osteotomy is made at the site of fracture. A wedge-shaped defect is opened on the lateral and dorsal aspects of the radius until the articular plane of the distal end of the radius is restored to its normal inclination. The distal prominence of the ulna is then removed with an osteotome and forced into the open wedge to maintain the reduction. A plaster cast should be worn for six weeks.

FLEXION FRACTURES

The distal fragment in reversed Colles' fractures is displaced volarward and proximally. This type of fracture is much less common than the hyperextension injury. The deformity is less

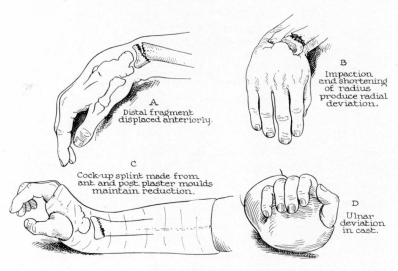

A
Distal fragment
displaced anteriorly.

B
Impaction
and shortening
of radius
produce radial
deviation.

C
Cock-up splint made from
ant. and post. plaster moulds
maintain reduction.

D
Ulnar
deviation
in cast.

Fig. 74.—The reversed Colles' fracture.

obvious than is the silver fork appearance of the hand and wrist after Colles' fracture. The principles of care are identical with those described for Colles' fracture. The final manipulation, however, should force the hand and wrist into moderate hyperextension. This cock-up position should be maintained by anterior and posterior plaster splints which are molded to the arm from just below the elbow to the wrist and include the hand to, but not beyond, the metacarpal-phalangeal joints (Fig. 74).

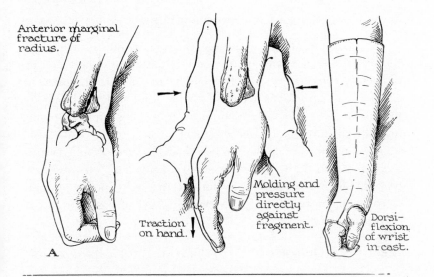

Anterior marginal fracture of radius.

Traction on hand.

Molding and pressure directly against fragment.

Dorsi-flexion of wrist in cast.

A

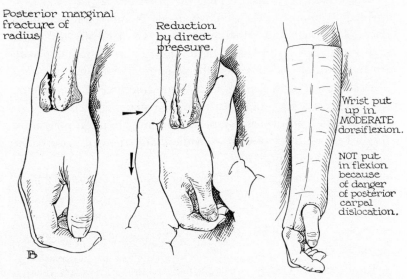

Posterior marginal fracture of radius

Reduction by direct pressure.

Wrist put up in MODERATE dorsiflexion.

NOT put in flexion because of danger of posterior carpal dislocation.

B

FIG. 75.—Fractures of the articular margins of the distal end of the radius.

169

Marginal Fracture

Anterior or posterior marginal fractures of the distal end of the radius are not difficult to reduce, but they should not be neglected or treated with indifference. The fracture fragment in either instance includes a portion of the joint surface. Displacement is rarely marked. Reduction can be accomplished by molding and pressure against the fragment.

Both anterior and posterior marginal fractures should be immobilized with the wrist held in slight dorsiflexion. The posterior type should not be treated by forcing the wrist into a position of volar flexion because of the definite danger of posterior carpal dislocation (Fig. 75).

Fracture-Dislocations of Distal Radial Epiphysis

This fracture occurs through the zone of partially calcified cartilage columns on the diaphyseal side of the epiphyseal plate and not through the growth-disk itself. Occasionally the distal end of the ulna is displaced, either alone or in conjunction with the radial epiphysis. The medial collateral ligament may be torn.

Dislocations of the epiphysis, oblique fractures of the epiphysis which cross the epiphyseal cartilage plate and crushing injuries directed upward through the hand may result in premature fusion between the epiphysis and the diaphysis with disturbance of growth (Figs. 76 and 77).

CLINICAL APPEARANCE.—The appearance of the wrist following an epiphyseal fracture-dislocation may be similar to that of Colles' fracture. The distal fragment may be dislocated toward the radius or toward the ulna, with a varying degree of posterior displacement.

REDUCTION.—This is accomplished by the maneuvers recommended in the treatment of Colles' fracture. The manipulations should be carried out with skill and with as little force as possible so that additional damage to the columns of growth cartilage may be avoided. If these attempts through careful manipulation do not secure an anatomic reposition of the epiphysis, future growth may be expected to correct most of the dis-alignment. A fair reduction should be preferred to an ideal restitution of the fragments through forced manipulation or open reduction,

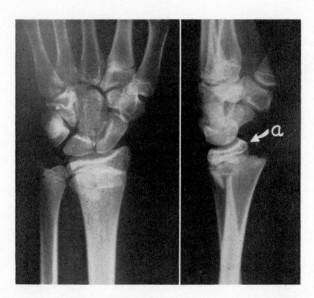

Fig. 76.—Typical epiphyseal fracture of the distal radial epiphysis with posterior displacement in a boy approaching puberty. The epiphysis, *a*, is displaced posteriorly from the metaphysis.

which greatly increases the hazard of arrest of growth from this center. The wrist should be immobilized for six weeks by anterior and posterior plaster splints, with the hand in a moderate degree of flexion and ulnar deviation.

FOLLOW-UP CARE.—Every case of fracture-dislocation of the distal radial epiphysis should be followed by roentgen study at six month intervals until the question of premature closure of

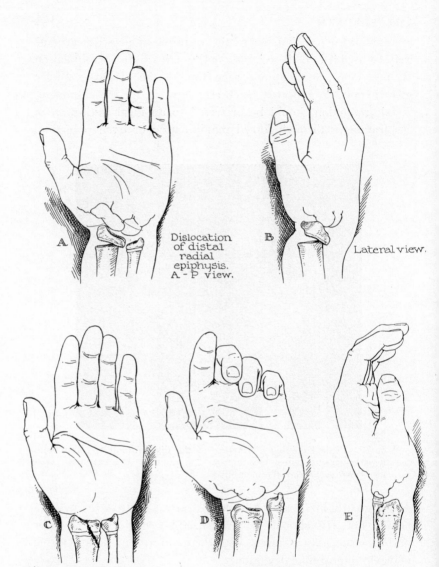

A   Dislocation
of distal
radial
epiphysis.
A - P view.

B   Lateral view.

C   Diagonal fracture across
radial epiphysis, growth
cartilage and cortex
of metaphysis.

D   E   Typical end-result after either
dislocation of distal radial epiphysis
or diagonal fracture if growth of
radius is arrested. Note continued growth of ulna.

FIG. 77.—Injuries of the distal epiphysis of the radius.

172

the epiphyseal cartilaginous disk is definitely answered. The parents of the patient must be forewarned of the possibility of growth arrest. When bony fusion occurs between the epiphysis

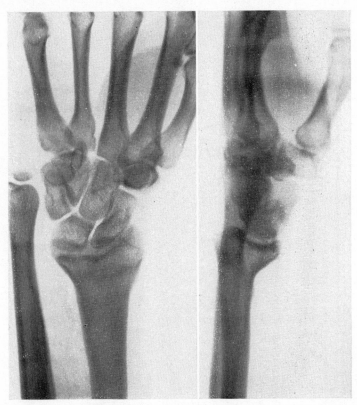

Fig. 78.—Marked shortening of radius in patient aged 19. Fracture at the age of 11 caused cessation of growth from the distal radial epiphysis. (Courtesy of Dr. C. H. Hatcher.)

and the diaphysis, it may be necessary to resect the growth zone at the distal end of the ulna to prevent overgrowth of this bone, with radial deviation of the hand and pain in the radial-ulnar joint. Resection of the ulnar cartilage is not indicated if the patient is old enough at the time of the injury to be approaching skeletal maturity and spontaneous closure of the epiphysis (Fig. 78).

If growth inequality is not prevented and deformity with pain

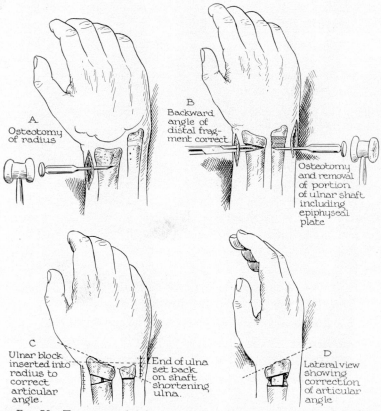

FIG. 79.—Treatment of deformity of the wrist caused by growth arrest of the distal radial epiphysis.

in the radial-ulnar joint persists, the distal end of the ulna should be removed to correct the deformity and relieve the pain and restore function of the wrist. A wedge osteotomy of the radius may be indicated (Fig. 79).

FRACTURES OF THE SHAFT OF THE RADIUS AND THE ULNA

These fractures will be discussed in the following groups: greenstick fractures in children, stable fractures of both bones in adults, unstable fractures of the radius and ulna, fractures of the radius, fractures of the ulna, fractures of the ulna with dislocation of the proximal end of the radius (Monteggia's fracture) and nonunion of forearm fractures.

The two bones of the forearm re-enforce and splint each other. The ulna is important in movement of the elbow and for stability of the forearm. The radius re-enforces the ulna, articulates with the carpi and makes possible the dexterity of the hand through its rotary motion about the ulna in pronation and supination.

The displacement of fragments following fractures of the forearm bones is dependent largely on muscle action and, to a lesser degree, on the force of the injury. The following muscles are involved, and the fracture surgeon must be familiar with their anatomy and function (Fig. 80).

1. The pronator teres, which has its origin above the elbow medially and inserts near the middle of the radius.

2. The supinator, which passes from the ulna to the radius posteriorly in the upper third.

3. The pronator quadratus, located anteriorly in the distal third, with its fibers passing transversely from ulna to radius.

4. The biceps brachii, which inserts into the upper third of the radius and serves as a supinator of the forearm and hand, in addition to its usual function as a strong flexor of the forearm.

5. The brachioradialis and brachialis are of lesser importance in producing deformity following fracture.

The nature of the deformity depends largely on the location of the break in relation to the pronator teres muscle.

A. When the fracture occurs proximal to the insertion of the pronator teres muscle, the upper fragment of the radius

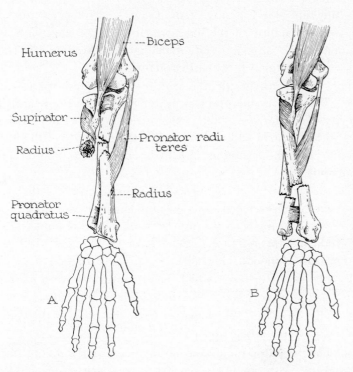

Fig. 80.—Schematic diagram of the forearm muscles which influence the displacement or rotation of fragments in fractures of the radius and ulna.

assumes a position of supination owing to the unopposed action of the supinator muscle. The distal fragments of the radius and ulna are pronated by the pronator teres and pronator quadratus muscles. The radius lies obliquely across the ulna, and for alignment of this fracture the surgeon must strongly supinate the distal fragments with steady traction throughout the maneuver.

B. When the fracture is distal to the insertion of the pronator teres, the proximal fragment of the radius assumes a neutral position, as the action of the supinator muscle is counteracted by the pronator teres. The distal end of the radius is pronated by the pronator quadratus muscle and drawn toward the ulna. Reduction is accomplished by obtaining end-to-end position of the fragments, with the hand in a neutral position between pronation and supination.

Oblique fractures usually result in shortening with overlapping of fragments. The interosseous membrane, with fibers passing slightly upward from the ulna to the radius, has a limiting effect on displacement of the fragments. Angulation at the site of fracture is usually posteriorly and is more common in the ulna than in the radius.

Recovery of dexterity and strength of the forearm and hand following fractures of the radius and ulna is contingent upon the preservation of the interosseous space and the restoration of pronation and supination. In general, the treatment of fractures of both bones of the forearm entails the following:

1. Restoration of length by traction on the distal fragments and countertraction on the proximal fragments.
2. Accurate apposition of fracture surfaces by manipulation.
3. Correction of alignment—both linear and rotary.
4. Restoration of the interosseous space.
5. Immobilization in a lightly padded plaster cast until roentgenograms show bony union. The elbow should be flexed to 90 degrees, and the cast should extend from the axilla to the distal flexor crease of the palm, but not to the metacarpal-phalangeal joints. The forearm should be fully supinated for fractures above the insertion of the pronator teres; and for fractures distal to this insertion, a neutral

position between pronation and supination should be maintained.

6. Oblique fractures which cannot be adequately reduced and maintained by closed methods must be treated surgically—by open reduction and application of plates and screws, insertion of an intramedullary rod in the ulna or skeletal pins above and below the site of fracture, with stabilization by a plaster cast.

FRACTURES IN CHILDREN

The shafts of the radius and ulna of young children are frequently broken by falls on the outstretched hand, while in adults such injuries usually cause Colles' fractures. The same type of injury may produce an epiphyseal separation if the patient is in the prepuberty age period of 12–15 years. The fracture in children is commonly located in the distal thirds of the bones. Often these fractures are incomplete or greenstick in nature with posterior angulation, but complete transverse or oblique fractures with over-riding occur. The greenstick fracture should be reduced by applying traction and countertraction, with correction of the angulation by molding the bone into line with the forearm grasped as in Figure 83, *B*. Care is essential to avoid loss of end-to-end position of the fragments. Excellent sedation and cooperation of the child may be obtained with an adequate dose of morphine, depending on the child's age. Do not try to inject procaine locally. The periosteum is not stripped widely, and it is difficult to locate a hematoma, which is essential for diffusion and successful use of this agent. Furthermore, the child will cry more during the insertion of the needle than during the actual reduction with adequate sedation by morphine. A long arm cast should be applied and check-up roentgenograms obtained. If the reduction is not perfect, the cast may be wedged, or removed and the manipulation repeated. The roentgen examination must be repeated 10–14 days after reduction since there is a tendency for angulation to occur as the swelling subsides and the plaster becomes loosened.

Fractures of the radius and ulna in children with separation and displacement of the fragments may be reduced by the same methods as those used for adults and will be discussed under that heading. If the fracture is transverse, the ends of the frag-

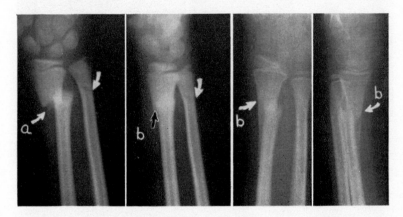

Fig. 81.—Open fracture through the distal thirds of the radius and ulna, *a*, in a growing child. Following reduction there was moderate displacement of the radial fracture but the position was accepted. Open reduction of a fracture of this type adjacent to the epiphyseal line is unwise. With the accepted position a normal functional result, *b*, can be predicted.

ments can be locked; but oblique fractures may occasionally require open reduction and internal fixation. Less than perfect apposition of fragments but good alignment may be accepted as an adequate reduction in a child, since callus is usually abundant and minor discrepancies are corrected by subsequent growth of the bone (Figs. 81 and 82). However, severe angulations may not be restored to alignment adequate for good function, and the physician must strive for as complete reduction as possible. If union is not complete at the end of six weeks, protection of the

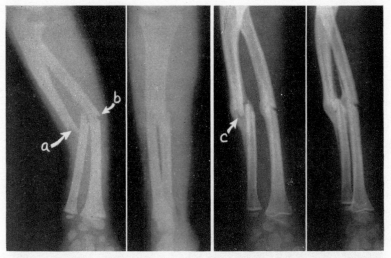

Fig. 82.—Closed complete fractures of the middle thirds of the radius and ulna in a child, 8. Marked displacement of the ulna, *a*, with angulation of the radius, *b*. Reduction of the ulna was not anatomic, *c*, but in a growing child, if immobilization is secure, union will take place and both external appearance and function of the arm will be normal.

fracture must be maintained by a plaster dressing for an additional four weeks or until roentgenograms show firm union. It is to be remembered that a small child will not understand what is meant by protected use of the arm, and refractures are likely to occur if immobilization is discontinued too soon.

Fractures of Radius and Ulna in Adults

When both bones are broken in the adult, over-riding and angulation are common. These fractures should be reduced by direct traction and countertraction. When strong distraction is required, traction with wire-meshed traps attached to all the fingers is eminently satisfactory. It is sometimes possible to combine gentle traction with marked angulation to lock the fragments of one or both of the bones and then to complete the

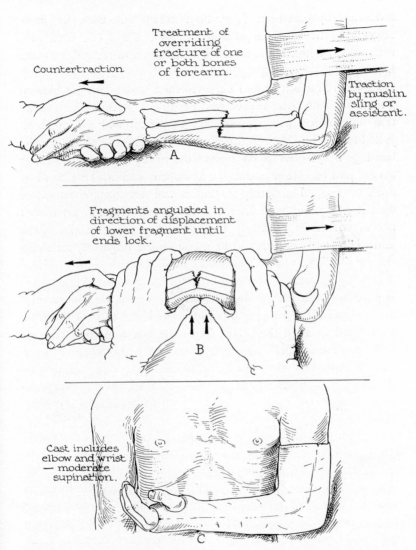

Countertraction

Treatment of
overriding
fracture of one
or both bones
of forearm.

Traction
by muslin
sling or
assistant.

A

Fragments angulated in
direction of displacement
of lower fragment until
ends lock.

B

Cast includes
elbow and wrist
— moderate
supination.

C

FIG. 83.—Skeletal traction or open reduction and plating should be used
if attempts to reduce by manipulation do not succeed in securely locking at
least the radial fragments.

181

reduction by extension (Fig. 83). When one bone has been aligned by traction, angulation or both, it may be used as a fulcrum for longitudinal leverage with which to reduce the other bone.

Closed reduction should be performed under local or general anesthesia. The latter is preferred because it permits total relaxation of muscles, which is difficult to obtain with procaine injected locally into the fracture sites. For countertraction, a muslin bandage may be wrapped around the arm just above the elbow over a pad of cotton batting or absorbent cotton. This bandage must be applied smoothly so that it will not become narrowed by wrinkling and with its sharp edges constrict the arteries or nerves which lie relatively unprotected just above the elbow joint. Direct traction should be made on the fingers by an assistant, or the fingers and thumb may be supported to an overhead bar by finger traps at the same time that downward traction is applied through the muslin sling. This permits the operator to use both hands as he attempts to interlock the ends of the fragments and to align the bones. With the bones in fixed traction and countertraction, a roentgenogram can be obtained to determine if reduction has been accomplished before the application of the cast. If the fragments are not reduced, the fracture must be remanipulated until the surgeon is satisfied with the reduction obtained.

A plaster dressing should be applied with padding of felt or cotton batting placed over the bony prominences of the condyles of the humerus and the olecranon. The pad placed under the sling on the arm during the reduction need not be removed. Anterior and posterior plaster splints, a circular cast or a combination of splints followed by circular plaster is recommended. The cast should not be extended as far as the metacarpal-phalangeal joints posteriorly or the distal palmar crease anteriorly, as it would then hinder free motion of the fingers and thumb. It should reach almost to the axilla, with the elbow flexed 90 degrees and with proper pronation and supination of the forearm. After the plaster becomes set, the sling around the arm may be pulled out of the cast. *It is absurd to attempt to immobilize fractures of this type with short splints,* which neither include the elbow joint nor prevent motion between the radius and the ulna at the wrist.

POSTREDUCTION CARE.—Few fractures have a greater tendency to displace than do those of the forearm. Loss of reduction may occur after a snugly fitting cast has been applied. A roentgenogram should be obtained after application of the cast and again after 10 days. If displacement or angulation develops and cannot be corrected by wedging, the plaster should be removed and the reduction repeated. The arm should be kept elevated and exercises of the fingers, thumb and shoulder started at once and repeated frequently throughout each day. Pain out of proportion to the initial trauma and associated with cyanosis or pallor of the fingers is a danger sign requiring immediate attention. Unless the circulation improves promptly and pain subsides, the plaster cast should be cut along its dorsal surface from one end to the other. *It is not enough to cut through the plaster.* Stockinet or sheet wadding or any other type of material beneath the plaster must be cut through also until the skin is exposed from the hand to above the elbow. When the initial swelling has subsided and circulation in the fingers is again satisfactory, the spread of the cast may be closed with circular plaster bandages.

If, in spite of opening the cast, the circulation does not improve, the possibility of impending Volkmann's ischemic paralysis must be considered and the cast should be removed until the condition is clarified.

Fractures of one or both bones of the forearm frequently result in nonunion, not because of a constitutional deficiency or because the reduction was not well carried out but because the immobilization was not complete or not maintained for a long enough time. Whereas union is usually adequate in six weeks in children, it may be necessary to maintain the cast for three months or more in adults. The time for its removal must be left to the judgment of the surgeon, based on good roentgenograms taken in both the anterior-posterior and lateral planes.

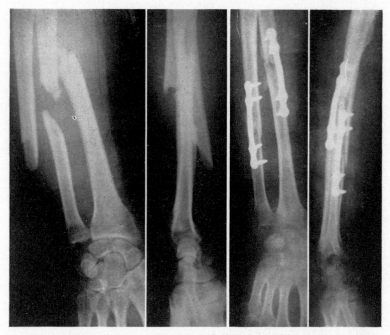

Fig. 84.—Fractures of the radius and ulna at the junction of the middle and distal thirds, with moderate displacement and over-riding. Because of the obliquity of the fractures, maintenance of position following closed reduction is difficult, and nonunion or malunion in fractures of this type are common. This fracture is best treated by open reduction and internal fixation.

Physical therapy is useful in restoring joint motion and muscle strength in adults, but it is unnecessary in children, whose joints mobilize quickly.

Unstable oblique or comminuted fractures of the forearm that tend to displace in the cast or cannot be adequately reduced by closed methods require operative reduction (Fig. 84). This may

consist of surgical exposure of the bones, reduction of the fractures and the application of metal plates fixed by metal screws.
Open reduction of both bones of the forearm is a difficult task
and should be attempted only by the experienced surgeon (Fig.

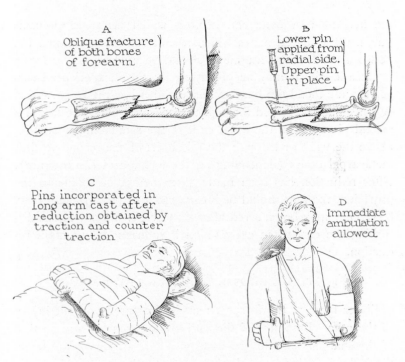

A
Oblique fracture
of both bones
of forearm

B
Lower pin
applied from
radial side.
Upper pin
in place

C
Pins incorporated in
long arm cast after
reduction obtained by
traction and counter
traction

D
Immediate
ambulation
allowed

Fig. 85.—Oblique fractures of both bones of the forearm are difficult to
reduce, and nonunion is common when less adequate methods of immobilization are used.

84). The ulna is exposed easily along its entire length by a dorsal
incision over the crest. No important structures are encountered
if the dissection is kept in this plane. The radius lies deep and its
exposure is more difficult. Open reduction for the radial head is
described in Chapter XX on elbow injuries. The shaft of the
radius is best exposed along its lateral surface through an incision

which parallels the anterior margin of the brachioradialis muscle
or tendon. Care must be exercised to protect the superficial
branch of the radial nerve and the radial artery. When metal
plates are applied to any bone, it is desirable to leave the periosteum attached along one surface of each fragment to decrease
the likelihood of bone end necrosis which delays or prevents
union. Only slotted plates which permit continued compression
between the fracture fragments should be used.

Occasionally it may be preferable for the inexperienced surgeon to use metal pin fixation above and below the fracture site.
A pin should be drilled through the proximal ulnar crest, and a
second pin through the distal ends of the radius and ulna 2 in.
above the wrist or through the midshafts of the second to fifth
metacarpal bones (depending on the location of the fracture).
After reduction has been made by a method available to the
physician, the pins should be incorporated in the arm cast (Fig.
85). They may be removed after six to eight weeks without disturbing the cast when early union is sufficient to maintain reduction.

FRACTURES OF THE SHAFT OF THE RADIUS

Either bone of the forearm may be fractured without injury
to the other. Fractures of the radius may occur in any portion
of the shaft and usually result from a direct blow to the bone.
Since the force is frequently directed from the lateral side of the
arm, the radius usually angulates or is displaced toward the ulna,
encroaching on the interosseous space. Reduction must be accurate in order to preserve normal pronation and supination. Closed
reduction may be attempted by strong traction on the thumb
and index finger and countertraction at the elbow. The bone
fragments should be angulated in an effort to lock their ends.
Open reduction and plating may be necessary, since closed reduction is difficult and often unsuccessful.

Fractures of the Ulna

Fractures of the ulna provide few serious difficulties in obtaining adequate reduction and union. The posterior and radial angulation may be corrected by traction and manipulation of the fragments. The arm should be placed in a long arm cast with the elbow in 90 degrees of flexion. There is a tendency for

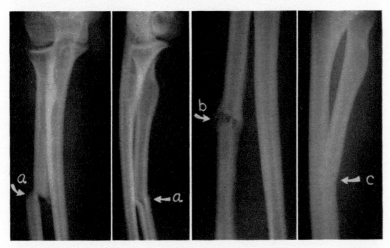

Fig. 86.—Closed complete fracture of the radius with moderate displacement and slight posterior bowing, *a*. The displacement is corrected by closed reduction, *b;* a satisfactory result is obtained with persistence of posterior bowing, *c,* due to muscle and interosseous membrane pull.

the forearm to angulate toward the radius and use of an intramedullary rod without a plaster cast has proved satisfactory. Union is usually firm in eight to 12 weeks. The elbow and wrist mobilize quickly, but this may be hastened by physical therapy.

Monteggia's Fracture

This injury consists of a fracture of the upper third of the ulna with dislocation of the head of the radius. If the fracture occurs

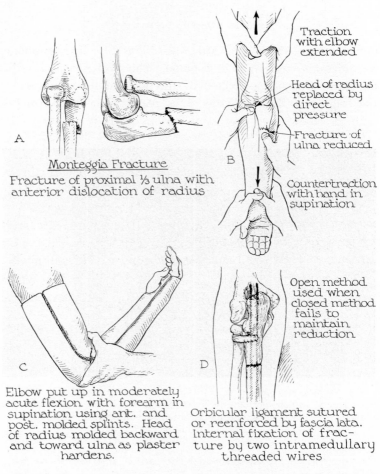

A

<u>Monteggia Fracture</u>

Fracture of proximal ⅓ ulna with anterior dislocation of radius

B

Traction with elbow extended

Head of radius replaced by direct pressure

Fracture of ulna reduced

Countertraction with hand in supination

C

Elbow put up in moderately acute flexion with forearm in supination using ant. and post. molded splints. Head of radius molded backward and toward ulna as plaster hardens.

D

Open method used when closed method fails to maintain reduction

Orbicular ligament sutured or reenforced by fascia lata. Internal fixation of fracture by two intramedullary threaded wires

FIG. 87.—Fractures of the ulna near the elbow with dislocation of the head of the radius.

with the elbow in flexion, the ulna angulates posteriorly and the head of the radius dislocates inferiorly with rupture of the orbicular ligament. Reduction may be accomplished by traction and countertraction with the elbow in 180 degrees of extension. The ulna rarely offers difficulty and the head of the radius can be molded anteriorly into position as a long arm cast is applied

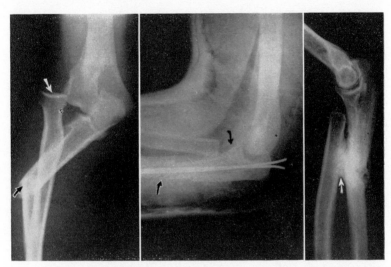

Fig. 88.—Severe Monteggia fracture of the ulna with complete dislocation of the proximal head of the radius, unreduced for four weeks when first examined. The head of the radius was excised and the fracture of the ulna reduced and immobilized with two intramedullary threaded wires. Subsequent bony ankylosis occurred between the radius and ulna at the fracture site. This is a disabling complication.

with the elbow in full extension. After union of the ulna is obtained, the cast should be removed and motion resumed.

The more common type of Monteggia's fracture consists of a volar angulation of the ulna with the head of the radius dislocated anteriorly. The fracture may be reduced as illustrated in Figure 87. The dislocation of the radius should be replaced by manual pressure over the bone and the extremity immobilized with the elbow in flexion. Open reduction of the ulna and insertion of intramedullary pins for secure fixation is frequently indicated and is preferable to the use of a plate. Cross union occasionally occurs and is a serious complication (Fig. 88). It is best not to perform an open reduction for the radial dislocation if it can be reduced and maintained by closed methods.

NONUNION OF FRACTURES OF THE FOREARM

If fractures of either or both of the bones of the forearm fail to unite following protracted immobilization, union can usually be obtained with an autogenous bone graft from the tibia. The graft serves as a splint as well as an osteogenetic agent (Fig. 98). The graft is fixed to the radius by screws. An intramedullary rod or pins will maintain alignment of the ulna, while an onlay bone graft will stimulate union.

CHAPTER XX

The Elbow

INJURIES of the elbow will be discussed
under the following headings: strains and contusions; epicondylitis; radial-humeral bursitis; dislocation; fractures of the head
and neck of the radius; fractures of the capitellum; fractures of
the olecranon; avulsion of the triceps tendon; supracondylar
fractures of the humerus; comminuted fractures of the distal
end of the humerus; fractures of the lateral condyle in children,
and avulsion of the medial epicondyle.

The elbow is formed by the articulation of three bones:
radius, ulna and humerus (Fig. 89). Besides flexion and extension motion at the elbow, there is rotary motion of the radius
which makes supination and pronation of the forearm possible.
Numerous ligamentous and bony injuries occur in and around
the elbow joint. Only the most frequent and important of these
will be considered in this chapter.

STRAINS AND CONTUSIONS

These occur most often in children. They may result from
falling or from twisting or hyperextending the arm at the elbow
as often happens in wrestling or playing football. The strain may
result in partial tearing of a portion of the capsule or the cap-

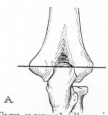

A

When normal elbow is extended the olecranon and epicondyles form 3 points in straight line.

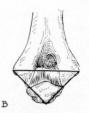

B

When normal elbow is bent the 3 points describe an equilateral triangle.

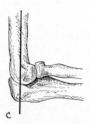

C

In lateral view the olecranon falls in vertical line with epicondyles.

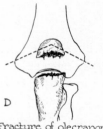

D

Fracture of olecranon distorts straight line.

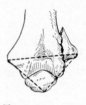

E

Fracture of lateral condyle distorts equilateral triangle

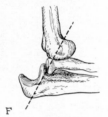

F

Vertical line distorted in posterior dislocation.

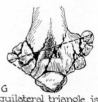

G

Equilateral triangle is distorted in comminuted fracture of distal end of humerus.

H

Normal triangle not altered in supracondylar fracture, but all displaced posteriorly and forearm appears shortened.

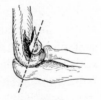

I

Condylar fracture with ant. displacement distorts vertical line.

FIG. 89.—Normal relationships of the medial and lateral epicondyles of the humerus and olecranon and their alterations in various types of fractures and dislocations around the elbow joint.

sular ligaments. It is followed by varying degrees of swelling which may produce synovial thickening and lameness that will persist for many weeks. After protecting the arm by a sling or a posterior molded splint for about two weeks, the patient should be encouraged to use the arm, but not to excess. Forced motion or stretching will only retard recovery and should never be permitted.

EPICONDYLITIS

In the adult, a common chronic traumatic lesion in the region of the elbow is that which has become known as the *tennis elbow*. This is probably the result of repeated forced pronation and supination and simultaneous firm grasping with the hand. The pathologic process is not well understood, but it is most likely a periostitis of the external epicondylar ridge. There may be an injury of the lateral ligament or common origin of the extensor muscles of the wrist.

The SYMPTOMS vary according to the acuteness of the underlying process. They may be so severe as to incapacitate the patient. Besides painful and limited flexion, extension and rotatory motion of the forearm, there are local swelling and exquisite tenderness along the lateral epicondylar ridge.

TREATMENT may be conservative or surgical. Injection of a 1 per cent solution of procaine into the tender area, together with rest by means of a splint, application of local heat and light massage, may effect a cure. Surgical stripping of the epicondyle may succeed when conservative treatment has failed. Even though no definite pathologic process is recognized at operation, the fibrous repair in the operative scar and the general healing reaction seem sufficient to mend the obscure lesion.

RADIAL-HUMERAL BURSITIS

This condition is the most common cause of pain and disability around the elbow joint. It is rarely correctly diagnosed.

SYMPTOMS.—Characteristically the patient complains of a toothache-like pain over the lateral side of the joint. This pain may radiate up the arm, down into the forearm or across the elbow joint and may be misdiagnosed acute arthritis. On examination the patient may be reluctant to move the elbow, and the pain can be reproduced by pressure on a very small, localized, tender (and sometimes swollen) area in the soft tissues along the lateral margin of the radial head. The *location* differentiates bursitis from epicondylitis, although both conditions may be present in the same patient.

TREATMENT.—Injection of 3 to 5 cc. of a 1 per cent solution of procaine into the tender area at weekly intervals may effect a cure after two or three treatments. The patient should be told to keep the arm at rest for 48 hours after each injection for the local pain is first increased after the effect of the anesthetic wears off. A patient with bilateral radial-humeral bursitis recently came to us for treatment. He had been unable to work for six weeks and had had his teeth and tonsils removed under a mistaken diagnosis of arthritis. He was relieved by one injection of procaine and was able to return to his job as a tuckpointer three days later.

DISLOCATION OF THE ELBOW

Dislocation of the elbow occurs most frequently in children and is usually in the posterior direction because of the hypermobility of the joint and the small size of the developing cartilaginous coronoid process. In adults, the displacement is usually associated with a fracture of the coronoid process. Lateral dislocation is rare because of the strong collateral ligaments and the broad articular surface of the distal end of the humerus. Most dislocations include backward displacement of both forearm bones, although either may be dislocated. Anterior dislocation of the radius occurs after rupture of the orbicular ligament or in fracture of the proximal third of the ulna (Monteggia's fracture).

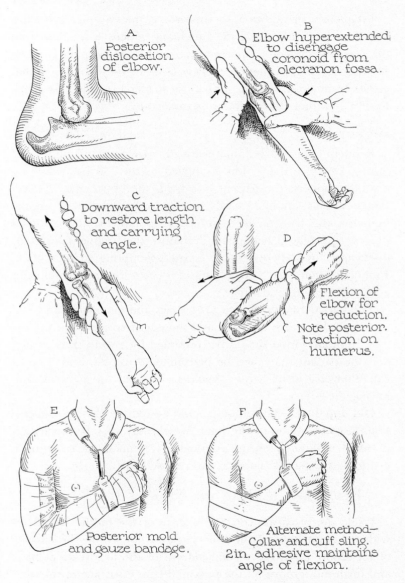

A
Posterior
dislocation
of elbow.

B
Elbow hyperextended
to disengage
coronoid from
olecranon fossa.

C
Downward traction
to restore length
and carrying
angle.

D
Flexion of
elbow for
reduction.
Note posterior
traction on
humerus.

E
Posterior mold
and gauze bandage.

F
Alternate method—
Collar and cuff sling.
2 in. adhesive maintains
angle of flexion.

FIG. 90.—Posterior dislocation of the elbow.

Frequently in addition to rupture of the capsule, ligaments and adjacent soft tissues, the brachialis anticus is avulsed from the coronoid process, a portion of which may be pulled off by the muscle. The formation of new bone in the hematoma that results from injury to the subperiosteal blood vessels may block flexion and limit elbow motion permanently.

REDUCTION

Reduction should be obtained with care to avoid additional injury. Downward traction is applied to the forearm while an assistant supports the patient and holds the upper arm. Reduction is usually obtained easily as the forearm is flexed on the humerus and traction is continued (Fig. 90). If the coronoid process is displaced behind the humerus, the fragments must be disengaged by hyperextension before attempting manipulation. Immobilization may be by means of a posterior molded splint or adhesive dressing and sling.

The patient should be urged to open and close the hand vigorously and to move the wrist and shoulder frequently during the day. Immobilization should be continued for two to three weeks, and the patient may then be permitted to use the arm. Forced extension or a lifting strain should be avoided for six weeks following the injury.

Old unreduced dislocations should be reduced by open operation. Reconstruction of the joint, which may vary from excision of small malunited or intra-articular fragments to a complete arthroplasty, may be necessary to restore function.

FRACTURES OF HEAD AND NECK OF THE RADIUS

While the proximal concave surface of the radius articulates with the capitellum of the humerus and lies within the capsule of the elbow joint, the medial margin of the head rotates back and forth in a groove on the proximal lateral surface of the ulna during pronation and supination of the forearm. Fractures involving the radial head and neck must be interpreted and treated according to the extent of functional disability which may be expected in the elbow and the radial-ulnar joint. These fractures usually result from a blow directed upward through the forearm, jamming the radial head against the distal end of the humerus.

CLINICAL PICTURE.—The patient complains of pain in the lateral aspect of the elbow. Examination reveals local tenderness over the head of the radius, limited motion, swelling of the elbow and pain on attempted supination of the forearm.

ROENTGENOGRAMS will demonstrate the exact nature of the fracture and will facilitate the decision as to whether conservative or surgical treatment should be instituted.

TYPES.—Fractures of the proximal end of the radius may be divided into four groups: (1) fissure, (2) marginal, (3) comminuted fractures of the head, and (4) fractures of the neck, with resulting impaction and tilting or complete displacement of the proximal fragment (Fig. 91).

Fissure or stellate fractures, which actually amount to cracks across the bone, are treated by a posterior plaster splint with the forearm in full supination for 10 to 14 days, followed by gradual resumption of function. If the reaction in the joint is minimal, the use of a sling with early motion facilitates complete recovery.

Marginal or "pie-crust" fractures involving a small area of the lateral circumference of the head may also be treated conservatively. On the other hand, a marginal fracture facing the radial-ulnar joint or the loss of a sufficiently large segment to interfere with function of the radial-humeral joint should be treated by excision of the radial head.

Comminuted fractures with displacement of fragments into the elbow joint can be adequately treated only by surgical removal of the remaining portion of the head in addition to the loose fragments.

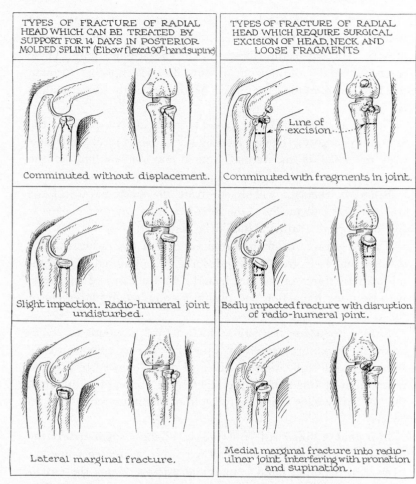

TYPES OF FRACTURE OF RADIAL HEAD WHICH CAN BE TREATED BY SUPPORT FOR 14 DAYS IN POSTERIOR MOLDED SPLINT (Elbow flexed 90°-hand supine)	TYPES OF FRACTURE OF RADIAL HEAD WHICH REQUIRE SURGICAL EXCISION OF HEAD, NECK AND LOOSE FRAGMENTS
Comminuted without displacement.	Comminuted with fragments in joint.
Slight impaction. Radio-humeral joint undisturbed.	Badly impacted fracture with disruption of radio-humeral joint.
Lateral marginal fracture.	Medial marginal fracture into radio-ulnar joint interfering with pronation and supination.

Line of excision

FIG. 91.—Choice of treatment of various types of fractures of the head of the radius.

198

Fractures involving the neck of the radius with slight impaction and tilting are treated conservatively. If the angulation is marked or the head fragment is displaced into the joint cavity

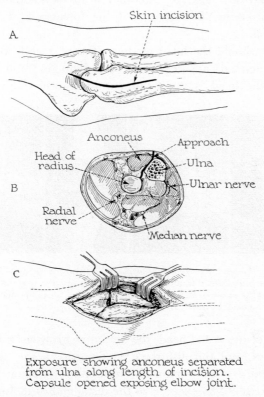

Exposure showing anconeus separated from ulna along length of incision. Capsule opened exposing elbow joint.

Fig. 92.—A safe exposure for resection of head of the radius. Too often the dorsal interosseous (radial) nerve is severed as it transverses the supinator muscle when the inexperienced surgeon places the incision directly over the radial head. This results in wristdrop which may be permanent.

or the adjacent soft tissues, so as to interfere with function of the elbow, the proximal end should be excised.

Whenever indicated, excision of the radial head should be performed as soon after the injury as possible. The approach is through a posterior incision, avoiding injury to the orbicular ligament and to the radial nerve as it traverses the supinator muscle in front of and below the proximal end of the radius (Fig. 92). The arm is immobilized for seven days, with the elbow flexed to 90 degrees and the forearm in a position of supination.

Rarely should the head of the radius of a child be removed. If the fragments are displaced, open reduction and reconstruction of the head is the treatment of choice (Fig. 93). After

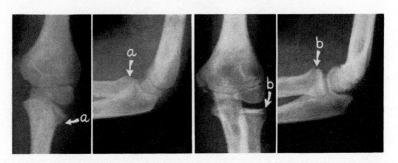

Fig. 93.—Impacted moderately displaced fracture of the head of the radius, *a*, in a boy, 5. Accurate reduction is essential to prevent permanent deformity of the carrying angle of the elbow. Open reduction is usually necessary, and in this patient normal growth from the epiphysis was preserved, *b*.

excision of the radial head, the ulna may grow to be longer than the radius, and the disturbed relationship in the distal radial-ulnar joint may cause pain and instability. Function of the wrist may be restored by excision of the distal end of the ulna, including the portion that contacts the radius, after the patient has attained skeletal maturity.

FRACTURES OF THE CAPITELLUM

Forces which are transmitted up the forearm may injure the capitellum. The injury may consist of bruising of the articular cartilage without an associated fracture. Greater trauma may displace small fragments of the articular cartilage from the capitellum, with varying amounts of the subchondral bone, into the joint. These fragments should be excised.

Large fragments which include a major portion of the capitellum and the trochlea should be replaced by manipulation, if possible. The fragment is usually displaced upward in front of

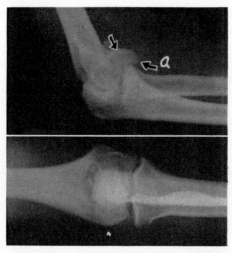

Fig. 94.—Comminuted fracture of the capitellum with typical anterior displacement, *a*. The capitellum is usually rotated and it may be impossible to replace in anatomic position by any closed method. Open reduction of the capitellum with internal fixation with threaded wires or screws is then the method of choice.

the humerus, and manipulation is carried out by a combination of direct traction with the arm completely extended and direct pressure to push the fragment down and back into normal position. Occasionally reduction may be maintained with a plaster cast which immobilizes the arm with the elbow flexed to a right angle. If the fragments are not securely locked, the arm should be immobilized in complete extension.

When an accurate reduction cannot be obtained by manipulation, the joint should be opened through an anterolateral incision (Fig. 94). All small detached bone fragments should be removed, together with the blood clots. The major fragment may then be examined and rotated into position. If a considerable amount of soft tissue attachment remains intact, the fragment may be expected to survive with a good functional result. If the capitellum and trochlea are both fragmented or if the major fragment is present as a free body in the anterior portion of the joint, completely or almost completely detached from the ligaments and capsule, an effort should be made to reconstruct the joint. Fixation is secured by pins or screws. Union may take place and although aseptic necrosis with absorption of the articular cartilage will almost certainly follow, the elbow will be stable and relatively pain-free.

Fractures of the Olecranon

The olecranon process of the ulna is more exposed to injury than is any other bone in the region of the elbow. The function of the olecranon process is to aid in maintaining stability of the joint. It also serves as a lever to the end of which is attached the tendon of the triceps muscle. Most fractures of the olecranon result from a fall. If the fracture is incomplete and there is no displacement of any fragment, adequate immobilization can be obtained by use of a posterior molded plaster splint with the elbow flexed and the forearm in midpronation and supination. If the fracture is complete but with no separation of fragments, immobilization in extension is indicated (Fig. 95).

OPEN REDUCTION

If the pull of the triceps muscle produces and maintains separation of the fragments, open reduction is imperative. The elbow joint is approached by a posterolateral incision. The major fragment is retracted proximally and the joint carefully inspected. The blood clot and all small detached fragments are removed.

The major fragment or fragments are reduced by careful fitting
of fracture surfaces; immobilization may then be made secure
by inserting two threaded steel pins, screws or heavy steel wire
(Fig. 96). The pins are of stainless steel, gauge 0.093 (3/32 in.)
with 48 threads to the inch. They are sharpened to a drill point
and are inserted from just below the attachment of the tendon
of the triceps muscle in a direction parallel to the long axis of
the ulna. Two such threaded pins will hold securely, even

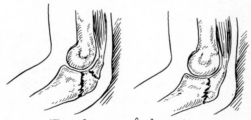

Fractures of olecranon
with minimal displacement.

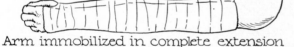

Arm immobilized in complete extension
with ant. and post. mold from wrist to axilla.

Fig. 95.—Fractures of the olecranon without displacement of the triceps
fragment may be treated with a plaster splint.

though they may pass through three or four separate fragments
before engaging the uninjured portion of the ulnar shaft. The
pins are cut off so that the ends will be covered over by the skin
and subcutaneous fat when the incision is closed. Excellent results are also obtained with internal fixation by means of heavy
steel wire. The wire should be looped through the triceps tendon
above and through the distal bone fragment below. The pins or
wire should be removed after the fracture has healed (Fig. 97).

A posterior molded plaster splint which extends from just

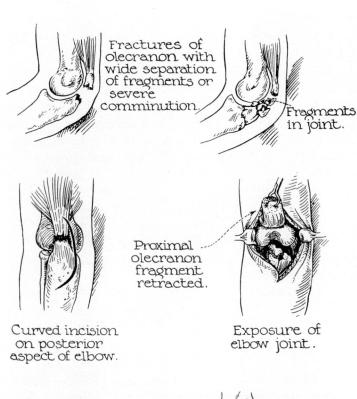

Fractures of olecranon with wide separation of fragments or severe comminution.

Fragments in joint.

Curved incision on posterior aspect of elbow.

Proximal olecranon fragment retracted.

Exposure of elbow joint.

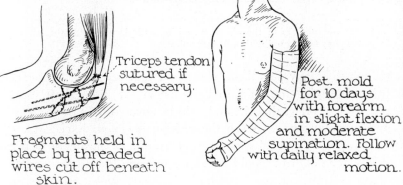

Triceps tendon sutured if necessary.

Fragments held in place by threaded wires cut off beneath skin.

Post. mold for 10 days with forearm in slight flexion and moderate supination. Follow with daily relaxed motion.

FIG. 96.—Most fractures of the olecranon require open reduction and internal fixation. We find the small threaded pins efficient in maintaining position of the fragments while permitting early relaxed motion.

204

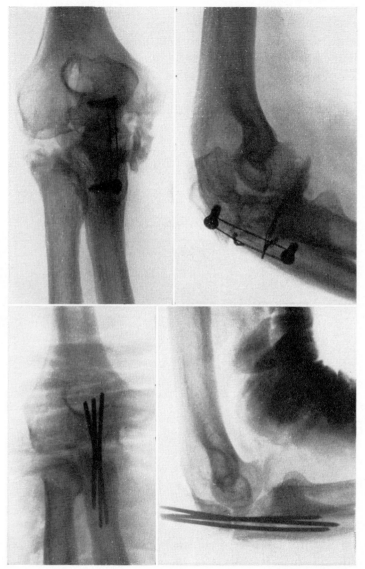

Fig. 97.—Use of threaded pins for internal fixation of the olecranon after removal of wires and screws and arthroplasty of the elbow. This patient obtained 95 degrees of painless motion with good strength and function.

proximal to the metacarpal-phalangeal joints of the hand almost to the axilla, with the forearm held in a position of supination and the elbow flexed 45 degrees, should be worn for 10 days. Active motion may be permitted afterward and *at no time should any stretching or forced motion be permitted.*

Old nonunion of the olecranon should be treated by open reduction, débridement of the elbow joint, osteoperiosteal or full

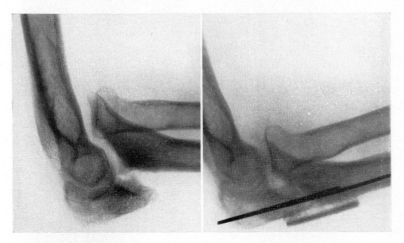

FIG. 98.—Ununited and unreduced fracture of the ulna with dislocation of the radius eight months after injury. Healing followed open reduction, onlay autogenous bone graft and internal fixation by two threaded pins. (Courtesy of Dr. D. B. Phemister.)

thickness onlay tibial bone graft and threaded pin fixation as illustrated in Figure 98.

AVULSION OF THE TRICEPS TENDON

Avulsion of the triceps tendon is a rare injury. When it does occur, all small fragments of bone should be excised and the tendon of the triceps sutured with no. 2 chromic catgut or fine wire to the fracture surface of the distal fragment. As much as half of the olecranon can be excised without impairing function. Motion may be resumed after 14 days.

SUPRACONDYLAR FRACTURES OF THE HUMERUS

Supracondylar fractures of the humerus may be associated with either anterior or posterior displacement of the condylar

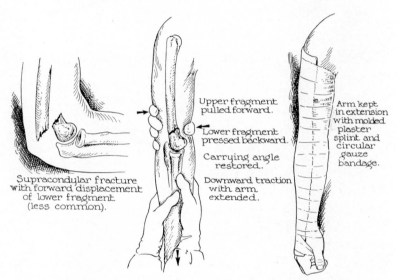

Upper fragment pulled forward.

Lower fragment pressed backward.

Carrying angle restored.

Downward traction with arm extended.

Arm kept in extension with molded plaster splint and circular gauze bandage.

Supracondylar fracture with forward displacement of lower fragment (less common).

FIG. 99.—Manipulative reduction of anteriorly displaced supracondylar fracture of the humerus.

fragment. Reduction is obtained by manipulation or traction and should be followed by frequent roentgenographic check-ups. When the distal condylar fragment is displaced *anteriorly,* reduction may be obtained by downward traction and extension and maintained in extension by molded plaster splints (Fig. 99). When the distal fragment is *posteriorly* displaced, reduction may be obtained by traction applied in the long axis of the limb, followed by flexion of the elbow. Position is maintained by means of a posterior molded plaster splint and a collar and cuff sling

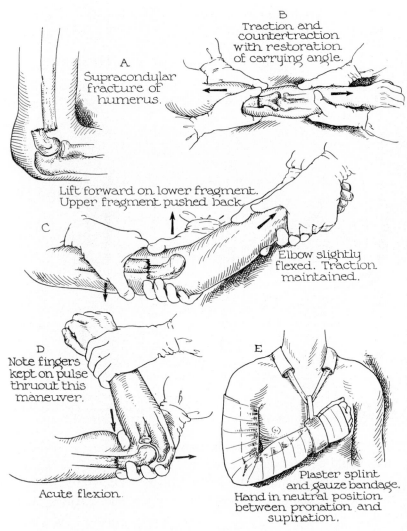

A
Supracondylar
fracture of
humerus.

B
Traction and
countertraction
with restoration
of carrying angle.

Lift forward on lower fragment.
Upper fragment pushed back.

C

Elbow slightly
flexed. Traction
maintained.

D
Note fingers
kept on pulse
thruout this
maneuver.

Acute flexion.

E

Plaster splint
and gauze bandage.
Hand in neutral position
between pronation and
supination.

FIG. 100.—Posteriorly displaced supracondylar fracture of the humerus.

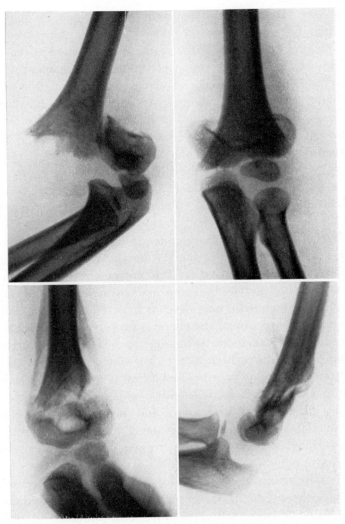

Fig. 101.—Typical supracondylar fracture of the humerus with posterior and upward displacement of distal fragment. The fracture was easily reduced by manipulation, but required continuous traction for two weeks because of displacement in plaster following reduction. There was normal function one year after injury.

(Fig. 100). If the fracture line is long and oblique, the hanging cast may be used without preliminary attempts at reduction of the fracture. The weight of the cast and the position of the arm will lead to gradual restoration of length and alignment of the humerus. In children, reduction is achieved by traction (Fig. 101).

While carrying out a manipulative reduction of a fracture in the region of the elbow joint and flexion is necessary to obtain or maintain reduction, the surgeon should check the radial pulse frequently. Compression of the brachial artery may result in severe circulatory injury to the forearm and hand.

Fractures of the distal end of the humerus in children may include one or more of the epiphyseal cartilage growth zones. The displacement may be both backward and to the lateral side. Such fractures are difficult to reduce. They should be treated by closed manipulation under general anesthesia (Fig. 101). Poor reduction of this transcondylar fracture or arrest of growth of the lateral condyle may lead to a marked increase in the carrying angle. Ulnar palsy may develop from 10 to 20 years later.

If the swelling around the elbow is excessive and prevents an immediate and adequate reduction, or if the distal fragment cannot be held in position in the cast, skeletal traction through the crest of the ulna may be used (Fig. 102). After the reduction, and when the swelling subsides (usually in 10 to 14 days), molded plaster splints are applied and the patient is allowed to be ambulatory. After six weeks, union should be sufficient, as demonstrated in roentgenograms, to permit removal of the cast and active motion of the elbow.

Accurate reduction should restore the fragments to a position in which the distal humeral epiphysis projects forward and down from the end of the shaft at an angle of 45 degrees (Fig. 101). The end-result should be complete flexion and extension of the elbow.

It is impossible to overemphasize the importance of observing the circulation of the fingers at frequent intervals for 48 to 72

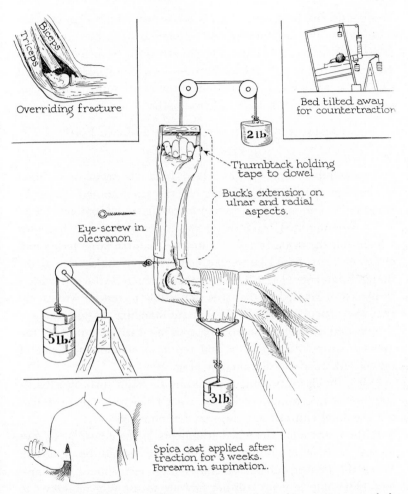

Overriding fracture

Bed tilted away
for countertraction

2 lb.

Thumbtack holding
tape to dowel

Buck's extension on
ulnar and radial
aspects.

Eye-screw in
olecranon

5 lb.

3 lb.

Spica cast applied after
traction for 3 weeks.
Forearm in supination.

FIG. 102.—Excessive swelling or obliquity of the fracture may preclude immediate manipulative reduction of a supracondylar fracture of the humerus. Continuous traction is the method of choice.

211

hours after the reduction. This is the injury which is most often followed by the development of Volkmann's contracture, which is brought on by obstruction of venous return from the forearm. Injuries to the radial and median nerves are not infrequent and should be recognized before reduction is attempted. Recovery is usually complete in four to five months.

COMMINUTED FRACTURES OF DISTAL END
OF THE HUMERUS

Transcondylar and supracondylar fractures occur more often in children than in adults, whereas the comminuted T- or Y-fracture is a more common injury of the older patients (Fig. 103). Comminuted fractures of the lower end of the humerus which split the distal fragment into two or three large pieces and enter the joint should be treated conservatively unless one of the major fragments or a portion of the articular surface is widely displaced or rotated so that it is impossible to restore with accuracy the articular surfaces. Use of the hanging plaster cast is a simple and excellent method of treating this fracture. Its use avoids manipulative trauma and results in a high incidence of union with good elbow function (Fig. 104).

When the distal fragment, including the joint surface, is badly comminuted, continuous skeletal traction, with a pin through the proximal end of the ulna, may be indicated.

If there are small detached fragments in the elbow joint, just as was true of olecranon fractures, they should be removed. When the joint is opened, all major fragments should be examined. The able surgeon will not hesitate to use pins or screws to hold large fragments securely in position (Fig. 105). The screws should not be inserted through an articular surface. A satisfactory approach to the distal end of the humerus may be secured through a posterior incision, dividing the triceps tendon in a manner which will leave a triangular, or tongue-shaped, portion attached to the olecranon.

Fractures of the Lateral Condyle in Children

The fracture line is usually oblique, starting on the lateral epicondylar ridge and extending down and medially into the

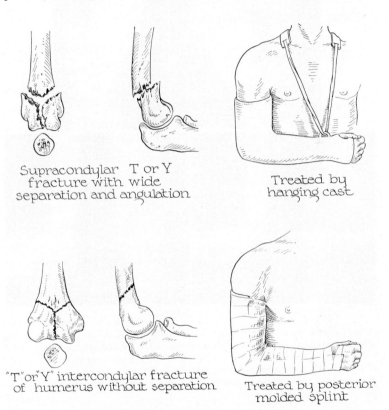

Supracondylar T or Y
fracture with wide
separation and angulation

Treated by
hanging cast

"T" or "Y" intercondylar fracture
of humerus without separation

Treated by posterior
molded splint

Fig. 103 *(above)*.—Supracondylar fracture with wide separation and angulation immobilized with a hanging cast.
Fig. 104 *(below)*.—T- or Y-intercondylar fracture without separation.

midportion of the joint. Usually, the fragment consists of the lateral half of the epiphyseal plate, a portion of the metaphysis, the entire capitellum and the radial extremity of the trochlea.

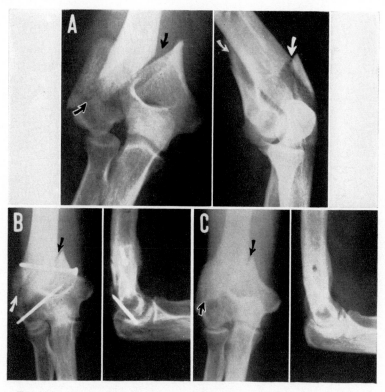

Fig. 105.—*A*, severe comminuted fracture of the distal humerus with several large fragments. Accurate closed reduction of this fracture is impossible, and open reduction is difficult. *B*, the large medial fragment was fixed to the proximal shaft with a stainless steel screw and the capitellum to this fragment with a threaded wire. Active elbow motion is encouraged as soon as early healing can be demonstrated by x-ray. *C* shows preservation of joint space six months after injury.

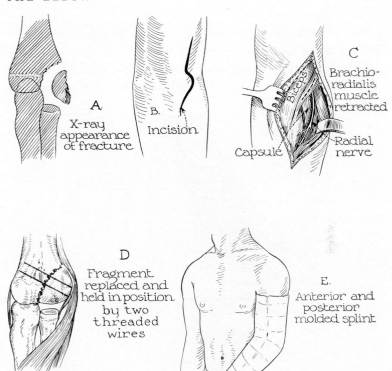

Fɪɢ. 106.—The capitellum fragment should be accurately replaced by open reduction and if necessary fixed by means of pins or screws.

Frequently the fragment is rotated laterally out of the joint through an arc of 180 degrees and flexed forward 90 degrees by the radial collateral ligament and the extensor muscles of the forearm. Because of this wide displacement, closed reduction is rarely successful, and in most instances open reduction should be carried out. Accurate replacement of the fragment is essential for restoration of good function (Figs. 106 and 107).

OPEN REDUCTION

The joint should be opened through an anterior lateral incision, avoiding injury to the radial nerve. The capsule is incised and the fragment replaced accurately into the defect at the end of the humerus. Frequently, the reduction is stable in moderate

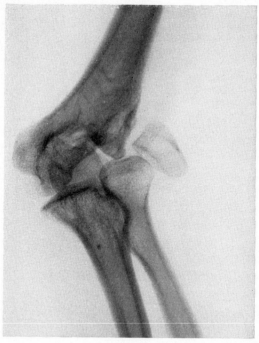

Fig. 107.—Old unreduced fracture-dislocation of the lateral condyle of the humerus of patient aged 31. Injury at the age of 2. There are deformity and late ulnar nerve palsy.

flexion of the elbow after suture of the soft parts. If the detached portion of the metaphysis is sufficiently large, it is advisable to fix the fragment with metal pins or screws, which are inserted in such a manner that neither the articular cartilage nor the epiphyseal plate is damaged.

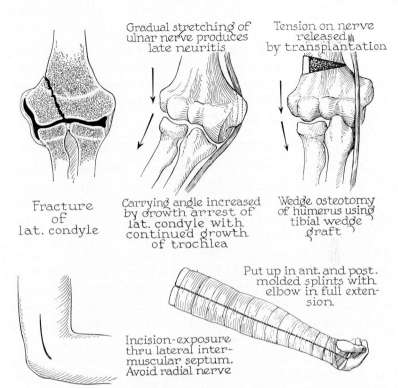

Gradual stretching of ulnar nerve produces late neuritis

Tension on nerve released by transplantation

Fracture of lat. condyle

Carrying angle increased by growth arrest of lat. condyle with continued growth of trochlea

Wedge osteotomy of humerus using tibial wedge graft

Put up in ant. and post. molded splints with elbow in full extension

Incision-exposure thru lateral intermuscular septum. Avoid radial nerve

Fig. 108.—Correction of deformity of the elbow caused by growth arrest of the lateral humeral condyle.

The parents of the child should be informed of the possibility of growth arrest with progressive lateral deformity, even though the reduction is accurate (Fig. 108). The late ulnar neuritis associated with asymmetrical growth of the lower humerus, following premature closure of the capitellum epiphysis, has been discussed in Chapter XIII.

Avulsion of the Medial Epicondyle

Forceful valgus strains or a blow to the outer surface of the elbow, with the flexor muscles of the forearm contracting, may avulse the medial epicondyle epiphysis of the humerus. This may occur at any age up to the time of closure of the growth plate, which is usually at about 17 years. The epiphyseal fragment may be incompletely separated from the shaft or displaced down to the joint level by pull of the flexor muscles of the forearm. If the valgus strain is sufficiently great, the medial collateral ligament is torn, and as the joint opens on the ulnar side, the epicondyle may be thrown into the joint and caught between the ulna and the trochlea, completely blocking elbow motion.

If the displacement of the fragment is minimal, the elbow should be immobilized for three weeks in a molded splint and then function gradually resumed. Displacement of the epicondyle to the joint level or into the elbow cavity must be treated by open operation and accurate replacement of the epiphysis for restoration of satisfactory function. In young children the epiphysis is small and largely cartilaginous. Because of the attachment of ligaments and muscles which pull it out of position, it must be fixed securely by means of some type of small wire or pin, even though this does produce additional trauma to the growth center (Fig. 109).

Accidents in which the arm is caught in power-driven machines may cause open fractures or fracture-dislocations of the elbow which challenge both the courage and the skill of the surgeon. If there is a pulse at the wrist, an attempt should be

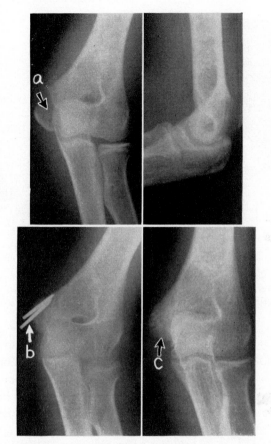

Fig. 109.—Fracture of the medial epicondyle of boy, 14, with moderate displacement, *a*. Because of the capsular attachments, this fracture is difficult to reduce and immobilize without internal fixation. Open reduction is relatively atraumatic and best results are obtained by this method, *b*. The threaded wires were removed when x-rays revealed union, *c*.

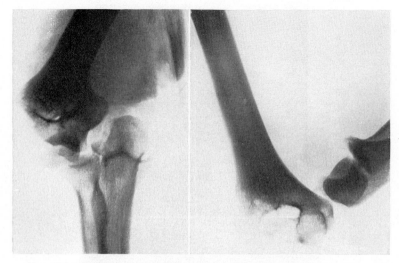

Fig. 110.—Open fracture-dislocation of elbow with almost complete avulsion of the entire forearm. Healed without infection after cleansing, débridement, reduction and primary closure, with recovery of function and sensation of the hand.

made to save the arm even though it has been almost completely avulsed at the elbow. Careful cleansing, débridement, repair of nerves and tendons, replacement of major fracture fragments and closure without drainage may lead to healing by primary intention (Fig. 110). The surgeon should not decide that it is impossible to save the arm and complete the amputation merely because he thinks the chance of saving it is too small to justify the effort.

CHAPTER XXI

The Humerus

$F_{RACTURES}$ of the shaft of the humerus may be transverse, oblique or spiral (Fig. 111). When the fracture occurs in the lower third or at the level of the lower and middle thirds, the action of the supraspinatus and the deltoid muscles will result in slight outward displacement of the proximal fragment. If the fracture occurs at the level of the upper and middle thirds, it will fall between the sites of insertion of the pectoralis major and the deltoid muscles. The pull of the pectoralis muscle will rotate internally and adduct the upper fragment (Fig. 112). Fractures of the neck of the humerus may result in marked displacement of the fragments. The proximal fragment will be abducted by the pull of the supraspinatus muscle, while the distal fragment is adducted by the pectoralis major and may be displaced up into the axilla by the combined action of the muscles of the arm and shoulder.

THE HANGING CAST

The hanging cast, first recommended by John A. Caldwell, is a simple and satisfactory means of treating most fractures in the humerus, other than the few which require skeletal traction, open reduction or shoulder spica casts. A long arm cast is ap-

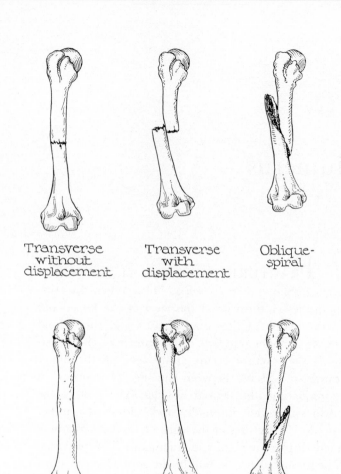

| Transverse without displacement | Transverse with displacement | Oblique-spiral | Comminuted |
| Impacted-surgical neck | Oblique-surgical neck-slight impaction | Oblique-distal third | Comminuted-distal third |

FIG. 111.—Fractures of the humerus.

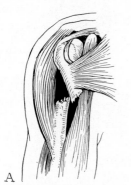

A
Fracture of humerus
below insertion of
pectoralis major.

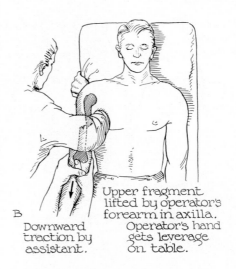

B
Downward
traction by
assistant.

Upper fragment
lifted by operator's
forearm in axilla.
Operator's hand
gets leverage
on table.

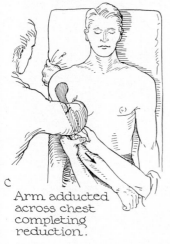

C
Arm adducted
across chest
completing
reduction.

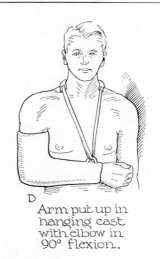

D
Arm put up in
hanging cast
with elbow in
90° flexion.

FIG. 112.—Fracture of shaft of the humerus between sites of insertion of pectoralis major and deltoid muscles.

223

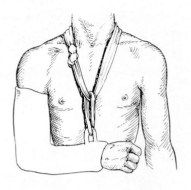

Hanging cast.

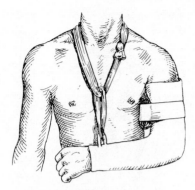

Felt roll in position
to correct medial
displacement of
lower fragment.

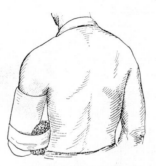

Sponge roll in position
to correct lateral
angulation.

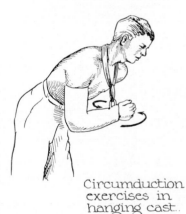

Circumduction
exercises in
hanging cast.

FIG. 113.—The hanging cast for fractures of the humerus permits daily exercises of the shoulder.

plied with the elbow flexed to 90 degrees. If there is marked
displacement of fragments, it is desirable to correct the displacement by manipulation under appropriate anesthesia. Roentgenographic examinations made in two planes at intervals of three
or four days following the application of this cast (which is
effective only if the patient is able to be reasonably active and
ambulatory) should show gradual improvement in alignment
and position of the fragments. If distraction occurs, the weight

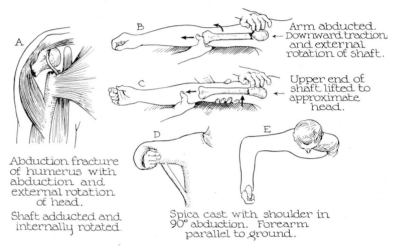

FIG. 114.—Fracture of the shaft of the humerus above insertion of the
pectoralis major muscle.

of the cast must be decreased. Angulation anteriorly or posteriorly can be corrected by adjusting the muslin bandage which is
attached to a plaster loop at the wrist and passed around the
patient's neck. Lateral or medial angulation of the fragments
can be corrected by attaching a pad of felt or gauze to the cast
to serve as a fulcrum for the arm as it presses against the side of
the thorax (Fig. 113).

This method of treatment has many advantages. It permits
immediate and continued exercise of the arm at the shoulder

and is far less cumbersome than the abduction splint or the arm and shoulder spica cast. The patient must be cautioned against sitting with the cast resting on a chair arm. This will defeat the purpose of the cast and may result in angulation of the fracture fragments. Night traction, that will both maintain reduction and relieve pain, may be obtained by incorporating a wire loop in the cast at the elbow. This is attached to weights through a pulley at the foot of the bed.

Within 10 days the patient should have painless free move-

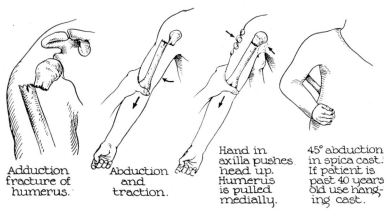

Adduction fracture of humerus.

Abduction and traction.

Hand in axilla pushes head up. Humerus is pulled medially.

45° abduction in spica cast. If patient is past 40 years old use hanging cast.

Fig. 115.—Adduction fracture of the humerus, just below the surgical neck.

ment of the arm at the shoulder. Use of the hand should be encouraged after the first week. Healing should be checked by roentgenograms after six weeks, and if firm union is not apparent, the hanging cast treatment should be continued for an additional four weeks. After removal of the cast, a collar and cuff sling should be worn for approximately two weeks, during which time motion and active exercises for the elbow, wrist and shoulder should be carried out daily under the supervision of the physician or a competent physiotherapist.

Fractures in the upper third of the humerus without marked

displacement may be successfully treated by the same method. If there is marked displacement, with outward angulation and rotation of the upper fragment, a plaster shoulder spica dressing, with the arm abducted and externally rotated 90 degrees, should be applied after reduction by manipulation or traction (Figs. 114 and 115). After six weeks there will be sufficient union to maintain apposition and prevent rotation. If necessary, a light

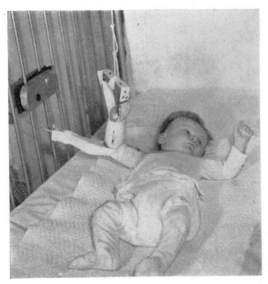

FIG. 116.—Simple adhesive traction for fracture of the humerus of an infant.

hanging cast may then be substituted for the shoulder spica cast, and exercise of the shoulder should be carried out each day. Subsequent care is identical to that described for fractures of the shaft of the humerus below the attachment of the pectoralis major.

SHAFT FRACTURES IN CHILDREN.—Closed fractures of the humerus in infants or young children may be treated by bandaging the arm to the side of the thorax. If the fracture is oblique, with over-riding of the fragments, lateral traction, using mole-skin adhesive, should be applied and maintained until callus can be demonstrated in the roentgenogram (Fig. 116). This usually requires about three weeks.

Skeletal traction is indicated in fractures of the humerus when there is marked comminution, with displacement of fragments

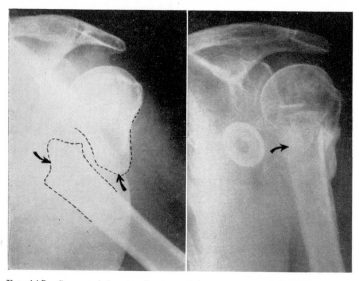

Fig. 117.—Severe abduction fracture through the neck of the humerus with displacement of the shaft into the axilla under the head. This fracture could not be treated by closed reduction. Following open reduction the extremity was immobilized in a shoulder spica cast for six weeks, when physical therapy was instituted.

which cannot be replaced by manipulation or reduced by a hanging cast. After reduction of the fracture, a hanging cast may be adequate to maintain alignment and length of the bone. Occasionally continuous skeletal traction must be employed, preferably with a threaded wire through the proximal ulna.

Open reduction is indicated when muscle tissue is interposed between the fragments and prevents reduction by either manipulation or skeletal traction (Fig. 117). A primary radial nerve palsy may be a second indication for open reduction.

Nonunion of the humerus is relatively uncommon. When it does occur, union may be obtained by a large tibial onlay graft fixed with metal screws. Immobilization by a shoulder spica or hanging cast is maintained until solid union is present, as indicated by roentgenograms.

CHAPTER XXII

The Shoulder

THIS discussion of injuries of the shoulder will be limited to the following: (1) fractures of the neck of the humerus, (2) fractures of the greater tuberosity, (3) simple dislocations, (4) dislocation with avulsion of the greater tuberosity, and (5) dislocation with fracture of the neck of the humerus.

FRACTURES OF THE NECK of the humerus may be impacted, comminuted or displaced. When comminuted, they are nearly always associated with fractures of the tuberosities (Fig. 118). When displaced, there may be moderate abduction and external rotation of the head fragment of the humerus. The proximal end of the distal fragment may be pulled medial to the head up into the axilla or the surrounding muscles. If the fracture is impacted, with minimal dis-alignment, a cuff and collar sling provides adequate treatment. Impacted fractures may show either abduction or adduction dis-alignment. If either is marked, there will be limitation of motion after union is complete. In elderly patients, the impaction should not be disturbed even when there is dis-alignment. In other age groups, however, if there is marked adduction or abduction with impaction, the fragments should be separated by breaking up the impaction by traction and manipulation. If, when the alignment has been satisfactorily corrected,

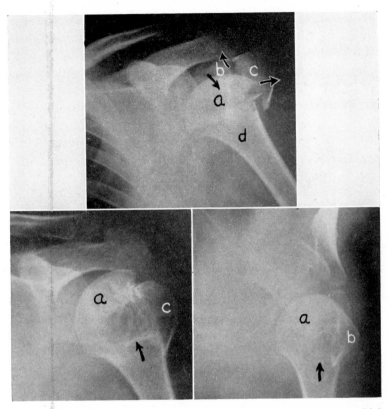

FIG. 118.—Comminuted fracture of the proximal end of the humerus which resulted from a fall on the lateral aspect of the shoulder. The head, *a,* has rotated laterally and distally 45 degrees so as to bridge the proximal end of the shaft fragment. The lesser tubercle, *b,* and the greater tubercle, *c,* have been displaced by the head fragment. Normal function of the shoulder resulted from an open reduction, despite aseptic necrosis of the head. (Note high density of head, *a,* compared to atrophic tubercles, *b* and *c,* and shaft, *d.*)

the fragments still interlock sufficiently to prevent displacement, a hanging cast or merely a wrist and neck sling usually maintains position (Fig. 119). An abduction frame or cast is much more cumbersome and is tolerated less well by the patient. End-results are often unsatisfactory because of pain and stiffness of the shoulder. Prolonged physical therapy is required in many

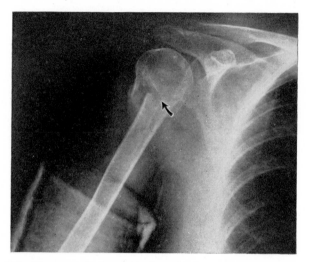

Fig. 119.—Fracture of the surgical neck of the humerus with moderate impaction, in our experience best treated by the use of a light hanging cast and early active motion.

cases to mobilize the shoulder, after which the pain will usually disappear.

FRACTURES OF THE GREATER TUBEROSITY of the humerus may be impacted without displacement, or the greater tuberosity may be completely torn away, with the insertion of the tendon of the supraspinatus muscle. A slight infraction or impacted fracture does not call for plaster immobilization. With separation of a major portion of the entire tuberosity, the arm should be maintained at 90 degree abduction and with the necessary degree of external rotation in a shoulder spica cast (Fig. 120). If the fragment is not reduced as the humerus is abducted, an open re-position of the greater tuberosity with fixation by a metal screw is indicated. After four weeks in a cast, the top half of the

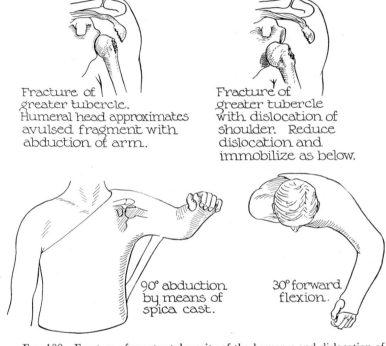

Fracture of greater tubercle. Humeral head approximates avulsed fragment with abduction of arm.

Fracture of greater tubercle with dislocation of shoulder. Reduce dislocation and immobilize as below.

90° abduction by means of spica cast.

30° forward flexion.

Fig. 120.—Fracture of greater tuberosity of the humerus and dislocation of the shoulder. The arm is abducted and externally rotated to replace the tuberosity after the dislocation is reduced.

arm and shoulder portion of the spica should be removed and the patient instructed in the use of the arm by lifting it out of the cast upward and rotating it both internally and externally. This program of exercises should be continued for an additional period of two weeks, when the cast may be removed. An abduction arm splint is then used while the arm is gradually brought down to the side. Only active exercise or relaxed motion is permissible. Any attempt to stretch forcibly before the eighth week may again displace the fragment which has not yet become firmly attached.

ACUTE DISLOCATION OF THE SHOULDER occurs most often in the anterior direction as a result of the abducted arm being forced into external rotation until the head of the humerus ruptures the inferior portion of the capsule and is displaced out of

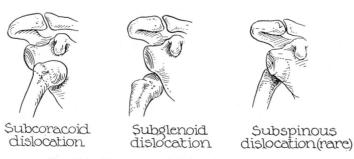

Subcoracoid   Subglenoid   Subspinous
dislocation   dislocation   dislocation(rare)

FIG. 121.—Three types of dislocation of the shoulder.

the glenoid. The dislocation may also be inferior or posterior (Fig. 121). Inspection of the patient with dislocation of the shoulder will reveal loss of the rounded contour, which is produced by the deltoid muscle as it lies over the head of the humerus and the upper end of the humeral shaft. If the injury has occurred only a short time prior to the examination, the patient will be in severe pain. He may be holding the hand and supporting the forearm, with the injured arm in slight abduction and forward flexion. Attempts to move the arm will be resisted. It will not be possible to place the hand of the injured extremity on the opposite shoulder.

Reduction of dislocation of the shoulder may be accomplished without an anesthetic. However, this is a severely painful manipulation, and an anesthetic should be given whenever a trained assistant is available to administer it. Pentothal sodium intra-venously is highly satisfactory. The manipulation should be per-formed without undue force, since a fracture of the neck of the humerus or additional injury to muscles or ligaments may result from forced rotation. The commonest position of the head of the

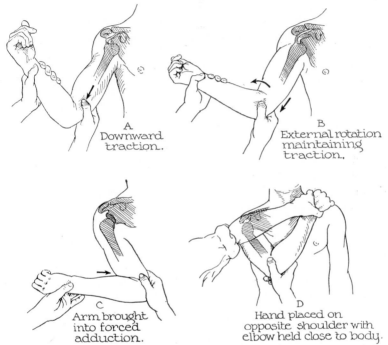

A
Downward traction.

B
External rotation maintaining traction.

C
Arm brought into forced adduction.

D
Hand placed on opposite shoulder with elbow held close to body.

Fig. 122.—Kocher's maneuver for reduction of anterior dislocation of the head of the humerus.

humerus is anterior to the glenoid fossa, and spasm of the sub-scapularis and pectoralis major muscles must be overcome to reduce the head of the humerus to its normal position.

KOCHER'S MANEUVER

The Kocher maneuver is most widely used and is a highly satisfactory method of obtaining reduction. The various steps are indicated in Figure 122. The patient is placed on a fracture table or stretcher cart, the wheels of which have been set in wooden blocks or braced with sandbags. The surgeon, standing on the side of the dislocated shoulder, grasps the elbow with one hand and the wrist with the other, maintaining 90 degree elbow flexion. Downward traction is made with the hand that grasps the elbow, and while this is maintained, the patient's wrist and forearm are moved slowly outward, externally rotating the humerus. *This is not forced, after resistance is reached, for fear of tearing the subscapularis muscle or producing a fracture of the neck of the humerus.* While the arm is kept in external rotation, the elbow is brought slowly forward in front of the chest and fixed there by the hand of the surgeon. The fourth step of the maneuver consists of internal rotation of the humerus by bringing the hand and forearm across the body toward the opposite shoulder. As the last step of this procedure is completed, the head of the humerus should slip smoothly into the glenoid fossa. If the tear in the capsule is very small, so that it constricts around the neck of the humerus, the procedure may have to be repeated several times before it is possible to tease the head back through the capsular rent.

Occasionally this maneuver fails. In such instances, direct traction on the arm should be applied in a downward and outward direction, while the surgeon produces counterpressure by placing his stockinged foot in the axilla. The right foot is used for a right shoulder and the left foot for a left shoulder dislocation. As the surgeon leans back and applies firm pressure with the foot against the ribs and the head of the humerus, the arm is gradually moved inward so that the foot not only presses the head of the humerus upward but serves as a fulcrum against the shaft of the humerus to pry the head out over the lip of the glenoid.

Direct traction will also reduce subglenoid or posterior glenoid dislocations. The subglenoid dislocation is frequently transformed into an anterior or posterior position by the first pull on the arm and is reduced from that position by direct traction and rotation or by the Kocher maneuver.

When the reduction has been obtained, a heavy cotton pad is placed in the axilla and the arm is bandaged to the side, with the hand resting across the chest. As in most injuries of the upper extremity, the hand and fingers (and, in this instance, the wrist) should not be immobilized. Active and vigorous exercises of the hand and fingers will greatly minimize stiffness in the rest of the arm. Immobilization should be continued for three weeks. When motion is permitted, it should be controlled active or relaxed motion only, such as swinging the arm in an ever-widening arc while the body is bent forward. For at least three months after the initial injury, the patient should not be permitted to engage in sports or other activities which may require a sudden upward reaching with the arms or to do any work which requires that the arms be held overhead. A second dislocation within a period of three months may produce sufficient relaxation of the capsule to be responsible for chronic recurrence.

COMPLICATIONS OF ACUTE DISLOCATION of the shoulder may include injury to any of the nerves of the brachial plexus, especially the nerve to the deltoid muscle. Transitory weakness and sensory disturbances may be present. Pressure of the dislocated head of the humerus on the axillary blood vessels can produce marked circulatory changes which require immediate reduction. Prolonged vascular disturbances of this type may lead to permanent damage to the structures of the entire arm.

Old unreduced dislocations of the shoulder require operative treatment. If only a few weeks have elapsed since the original injury, continuous skeletal traction or gradually increased traction on a fracture table, with the patient completely anesthetized, may obtain reduction. If the dislocation has existed longer than four or five weeks or if the attempt at closed reduction is unsuccessful, an open operation is indicated. The shoulder is exposed through an anterior deltoid incision. The coracoid process is osteotomized and reflected downward with the short head of the biceps and coracobrachialis muscle. This exposes the subscapularis muscle, which is retracted medially after its tendon is cut. The anterior capsule can now be opened and the head of the humerus exposed. An attempt is made to free the adhesions between the head and the glenoid. If reduction is not possible, the greater tuberosity is osteotomized and taken laterally to gain further exposure of the glenoid. Reduction can be effected as additional adhesions are released. The operation is concluded as the anterior capsule is repaired, the greater tuberosity sutured into place and the wound closed in layers. Active motion is allowed after three weeks.

DISLOCATION WITH AVULSION OF GREATER TUBEROSITY.— Avulsion of the greater tuberosity occurs in about one third of the cases of dislocation of the shoulder. Reduction of the dislocation is carried out as in the uncomplicated cases, but treatment must be administered with the arm held in abduction, external rotation and forward flexion (Fig. 120). We have no faith in the metal frames for maintaining this position. It is simpler to apply a shoulder spica cast, and the position is securely held. The patient will be more comfortable during the period of immobilization.

Recurrent dislocations of the shoulder are common and are likely to be seen in epileptic patients who suffer from grand mal attacks. Many operative procedures have been recommended for this condition. The Nicola operation has been widely used, although recurrences following this procedure are relatively high. The Bankhart operation repairs the torn anterior capsule and is becoming more widely advised. The pathologic anatomy varies, and combined procedures may be necessary in some cases to prevent recurrence.

FRACTURE-DISLOCATION of the upper end of the humerus constitutes one of the most difficult of all injuries to the human skeleton from the standpoint of obtaining and maintaining a satisfactory reduction. If the head of the humerus is dislocated and completely detached from the shaft, closed reduction of the dislocated head is exceedingly difficult. If attempted, manipulation should be carried out under sufficient anesthesia to obtain

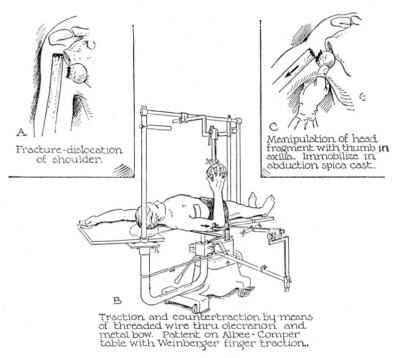

A
Fracture-dislocation
of shoulder.

C
Manipulation of head
fragment with thumb in
axilla. Immobilize in
abduction spica cast.

B
Traction and countertraction by means
of threaded wire thru olecranon and
metal bow. Patient on Albee-Comper
table with Weinberger finger traction.

Fig. 123.—Fracture-dislocation of the shoulder.

good muscle relaxation. An attempt is made first to reduce the fracture and produce locking of the fragments. This requires accurate determination of the position, including rotation of the dislocated head. The shaft of the humerus must then be pulled in a direction that will be in direct line with the longitudinal axis of the proximal or capital fragment. This usually means traction in an upward direction, with an assistant holding the scapula down. If the fracture fragments can thus be interlocked, it may be possible by continuing the traction to bring the head of the humerus back into position in the glenoid fossa. Immobilization may be maintained by bandaging the arm to the side in the same position as that used after reducing simple dislocations. If this position permits re-displacement of the fracture, as shown in the roentgenogram, it may be necessary to maintain traction with the arm abducted 90 degrees.

If the foregoing manipulation does not result in re-position of the humeral head and reduction of the fracture, skeletal traction by means of a pin inserted through the ulnar crest should be attempted (Fig. 123). As the proximal end of the humerus is pulled away from the glenoid, allowing space for the humeral head, an effort is made manually to manipulate the proximal fragment into the glenoid. In our experience, this is rarely accomplished.

Open reduction of the fracture-dislocation is imperative if all attempts to obtain reduction by closed methods fail. The anterior capsule is exposed as described under chronic dislocations of the shoulder, the head of the humerus is reduced and the fracture fragments accurately apposed and aligned. Fixation may be maintained by a loop of heavy stainless steel wire (Fig. 124) or a bone graft 5–8 mm. wide and 8–10 cm. long may be cut from the distal fragment, countersunk in the groove from which it has been cut and then driven upward into the head of the humerus across the fracture line. This makes an effective key for locking the fragments together and also aids in obtaining union of the fracture. It is best to discard the head fragment if it is comminuted or if satisfactory re-position on the shaft cannot be accomplished.

After open reduction, the arm is immobilized in a shoulder spica cast for four weeks. In an elderly patient, guarded motion may be started in three weeks with the arm held in position by a collar and cuff sling. Active use of the arm must be curtailed until there is roentgen evidence of union.

Complete fracture-dislocation of the head of the humerus may result in aseptic necrosis of the head fragment. This occurs following either open or closed reduction if the fragment is deprived

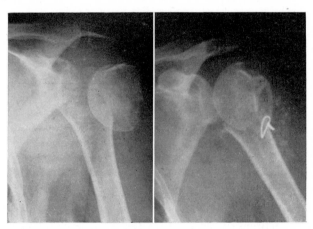

Fig. 124.—Severe fracture of the proximal humerus with anterolateral dislocation and rotation of the head fragment. Open reduction is usually necessary for adequate treatment.

of its blood supply. Union will take place in many of the patients and, since the replacement is usually without change in the shape of the head, prognosis is good. Mild secondary arthritis may cause some ache in the joint but the over-all function is better than when the head is excised. Excellent shoulder function is possible although roentgenograms are far from anatomic. Removal of the humeral head or arthrodesis of the shoulder may be indicated when there is nonunion or severe pain.

CHAPTER XXIII

The Clavicle and Scapula

Fracture of the clavicle or the collar bone has been too lightly considered by most surgeons. Malunion with angulation is common and nonunion is not unusual. Treatment by immobilizing the entire hand, arm and fingers, especially in older patients, has resulted in stiffness of the shoulder and sometimes of the joints of the hand and fingers as well. For a closed fracture of the clavicle, immobilization of the arm should rarely be necessary to maintain a reduction of the fracture. Fractures of the clavicle are most common in the middle third of the bone. The medial fragment is pulled upward and slightly posteriorly by the sternocleidomastoid muscle. The outer fragment is carried down and forward by the weight of the arm and scapula following the loss of its supporting mechanism. This deformity produces a shortening of the distance between the base of the neck and the tip of the acromion process. The deformity of an unreduced or a poorly reduced fracture of the clavicle may be particularly objectionable to a young woman who finds it conspicuous when she wears a low-cut dress. Strength of the arm and shoulder is diminished permanently by faulty management of this fracture.

Linear fractures without displacement are treated with a simple figure-of-eight dressing. With displacement and shortening, manipulative reduction must be obtained. Procaine infiltration is the anesthetic of choice. The shoulders are forced upward and back, and direct manipulation of the fragments is often necessary for end-to-end reduction. This position must be maintained during immobilization.

Following reduction, immobilization can be maintained in infants and small children up to 5 years of age by a figure-of-eight bandage. A pad of absorbent cotton is placed over the shoulder anteriorly and carried down into the axilla. The surgeon stands behind the patient and applies the bandage with some tension, wrapping it around over one shoulder, through the axilla (after passing it over the cotton pad), then up in such a manner that as he tightens the bandage he elevates the shoulder; then across the back over the top to the opposite shoulder, around the cotton pad and through the axilla and again up and over until at least eight to 12 turns have been made. This can be reenforced further with 1 in. strips of adhesive placed over the bandage and carried around the entire course of the figure-of-eight. While each turn of the figure-of-eight bandage is being applied, pressure should be made, either with the knee of the surgeon or by an assistant, over the spine between the shoulder blades at the base of the neck, so that the shoulders can be drawn backward as well as upward by the bandage. The one objection to this bandage is that it becomes loosened and migrates upward and must therefore be removed and re-applied every few days. The arms are left entirely free. When the patient sits or stands up the pad in the axilla serves as a fulcrum over which the weight of the arm drags, tending to maintain a distraction force in the long axis of the clavicle and preventing over-riding.

For the older child or the adult, a plaster of paris dressing should be applied exactly as the figure-of-eight bandage just

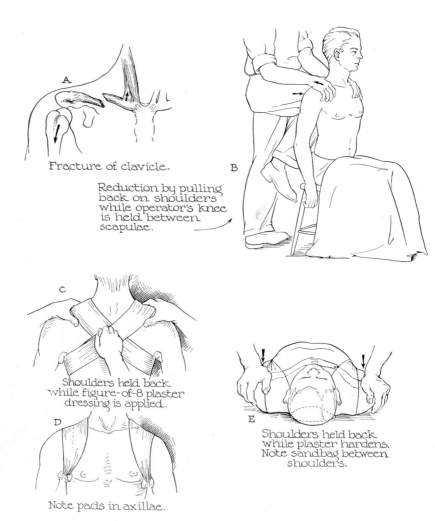

A

Fracture of clavicle.

B

Reduction by pulling back on shoulders while operator's knee is held between scapulae.

C

Shoulders held back while figure-of-8 plaster dressing is applied.

D

Note pads in axillae.

E

Shoulders held back while plaster hardens. Note sandbag between shoulders.

Fig. 125.—The figure-of-eight plaster cast dressing provides adequate, constant immobilization, permits immediate ambulation and free use of the arms.

described (Fig. 125). Beneath the plaster of paris a few turns of cotton batting bandage are placed around the shoulders in the form of the figure-of-eight dressing. Felt padding is required in the axilla and must extend beyond the edges of the plaster dressing. With the surgeon standing behind the patient, the plaster of paris cast is applied as is a figure-of-eight bandage, while an assistant pushes upward on the elbow and backward

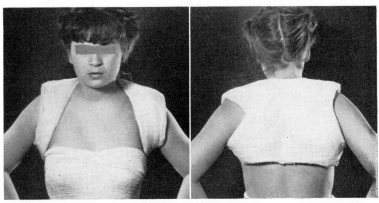

Fig. 126.—Figure-of-eight cast for fracture of the clavicle. Note the firm molding between the scapulae with plaster splints in the posterior view, as this is necessary for proper immobilization and stability of the fracture.

over the head of the humerus. The surgeon maintains pressure with his knee placed on the spine at the base of the neck between the superior-medial angles of the scapulae. At least 15 or 20 turns of plaster bandage 6 in. wide should be used. As soon as the dressing has been completed, the patient should be placed supine, with a thick roll of felt or a sandbag directly under the spine between his shoulders. The surgeon then applies firm pressure with the palm of the hand over each shoulder, forcing them back and up on the roll of felt. This will indent the plaster in the back where the bandages have crossed in the midline. The pressure must be maintained until the plaster has set and is strong enough to secure this position. While the patient is in the supine position, with the shoulders forced back and up, the arm should be brought as nearly to the side as possible. This method

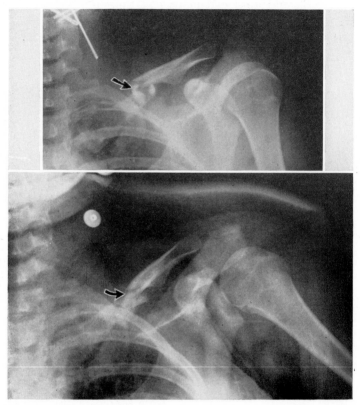

Fig. 127.—Closed fracture of the middle third of the clavicle with comminution and shortening. This fracture was treated with an ambulatory figure-of-eight plaster cast, with early healing and an excellent anatomic result.

can be used in the treatment of comminuted as well as of simple fractures (Fig. 126).

During the first three or four days after a figure-of-eight plaster dressing has been applied, the patient may suffer some discomfort from the pressure against the axillary vessels. This can be relieved at any time simply by abducting the arm and resting the elbow on a table or on the arm of a chair. After a few days the circulation usually adjusts to the pressure so that the initial discomfort in the arm is no longer present. Pressure must be relieved by trimming the cast if swelling of the arm is moderate or persists.

The period of immobilization varies with the age of the patient. Four weeks may be sufficient time to immobilize a fracture of the clavicle of an infant or a child under 5 years of age. Six weeks' immobilization should be sufficient for an adolescent or an adult, and a longer time may be necessary for the patient past 40. For all patients, immobilization should be continued until the roentgenogram shows definite osseous union (Fig. 127).

Children and adolescents quickly begin to use the arm on the side of the fracture, and little fear need be felt regarding a frozen shoulder. The middle-aged or elderly patient, because of pain or fear of pain, may hold the arm motionless at the side unless the surgeon emphasizes repeatedly the importance of actual functional use (not mere exercises) of the extremity during treatment. After about one week, if the patient has been cooperative, the arm will be surprisingly free from pain, and use of the extremity will be remarkably good for most purposes, in spite of the fact that both arms have been held in what appears to be an awkward position of abduction.

Open reduction is occasionally necessary. It is indicated when comminuted fragments are widely displaced or rotated and prevent adequate closed reduction. An intramedullary threaded wire is the best means for maintaining reduction (Fig. 128). After union is complete, the pin is removed by exposing the lateral end in the suprascapular region.

Ununited fracture of the clavicle is rare and is unlikely to occur if the fracture is properly treated from the beginning (Fig.

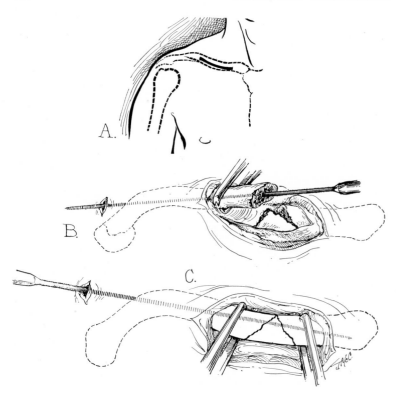

Fig. 128.—Intramedullary wire fixation of a comminuted fracture of the clavicle. The fracture site is exposed through a linear incision, *A*. A threaded wire is drilled outward through the medullary canal of the lateral fragment, piercing the cortex and emerging through the skin in the supraspinatus region, *B*. The fracture is reduced and the wire is drilled into the medial fragment, *C*. Other bone fragments are reduced and fixed by circumferential sutures of chromic catgut. The wire is cut off beneath the skin.

129). When nonunion is present and the alignment is satisfactory, it should be treated by open reduction and an onlay tibial bone graft. An intramedullary wire in conjunction with a bone graft is used to maintain reduction if the bone ends must be mobilized to re-align the fracture. Following this operation, a plaster figure-of-eight cast, as described, should be worn for 10 to 16 weeks, or until the roentgenogram shows good union.

DISLOCATION OF THE STERNOCLAVICULAR JOINT is less common than fracture of the clavicle. The acute cases may be treated best by the same type of dressing used and described for the treatment of fractures of the clavicle. If the figure-of-eight

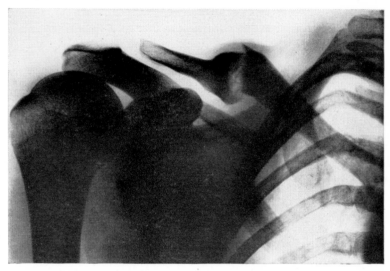

FIG. 129.—Old refracture of the clavicle with nonunion. Treated by open reduction and tibial bone graft.

dressing does not maintain reduction, a shoulder spica cast should be applied with the arm abducted to 90 degrees and in some degree of forward flexion and external rotation which offers the maximum reduction. If manipulative reduction cannot be obtained, open reduction may be necessary.

The ACROMIOCLAVICULAR JOINT may be dislocated with disruption of the coracoclavicular ligaments as a result of falls or other severe trauma such as may occur when tackling a runner in football. The injury is readily recognized by the downward displacement of the scapula together with the arm, the outer end of the clavicle being pulled upward. If the injury is confined to the acromioclavicular joint, the displacement between the clavicle and the acromion process is rather small with little deformity.

The presence of slight swelling, tenderness and local pain upon abduction of the arm should suggest the possibility of a subluxation of the acromioclavicular joint. Positive evidence of the degree of injury to the ligaments may be determined by x-raying both shoulders with the patient standing and holding a 20 lb.

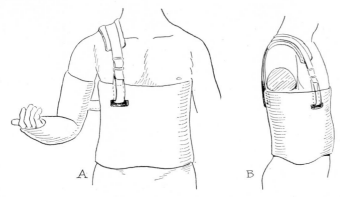

Fig. 130.—An effective conservative method for treating an acute dislocation of the acromioclavicular joint. The forearm cast is necessary for stabilization of the body jacket, effecting a steady corrective force on the clavicle.

weight in each hand. Many injuries of this joint go unrecognized and, without proper treatment, result in painful arthritis.

A satisfactory end result can usually be obtained by conservative treatment of the acute injury. The mild injuries can be treated in the following way. The arm should be supported by a sling which elevates the scapula. A pad of felt is then placed over the outer end of the clavicle and a firm adhesive dressing applied. The dressing starts on the back at the level of the waist and is carried upward over the outer end of the clavicle down to just below the bend of the elbow and back up onto the arm posteriorly. While the dressing is being applied, the arm is lifted at the elbow to elevate the scapula. The frequently used method of placing only short strips of adhesive criss-cross over the acromioclavicular joint is altogether inadequate for this purpose.

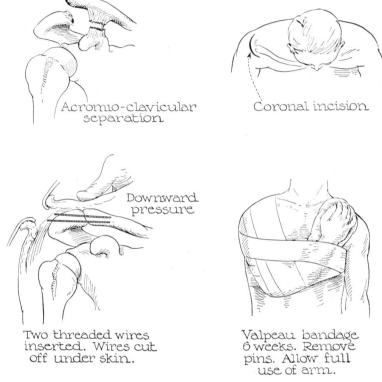

Acromio-clavicular
separation.

Coronal incision.

Downward
pressure

Two threaded wires
inserted. Wires cut
off under skin.

Valpeau bandage
6 weeks. Remove
pins. Allow full
use of arm.

Fig. 131.—Repair of acromioclavicular separation.

The best conservative method for treating the patient with high upward riding of the clavicle and complete rupture of the coracoid clavicular ligaments is shown in Figure 130. Considerable downward force is required, not only to reduce the dislocation, but also to hold it uninterrupted for the six weeks necessary for the ligaments to heal. The body jacket will ride up (and the corrective force be lost) if the arm is not incorporated as a part of the dressing. The patient will be temporarily incapacitated by loss of use of one arm, but this is a small inconvenience for a cure of the dislocation.

This injury is difficult to treat successfully. Constant supervision is necessary to insure optimal maintenance of the reduc-

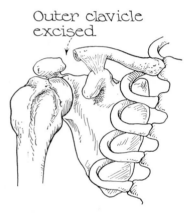

Fig. 132.—Mumford has demonstrated that dislocation of the acromio-clavicular articulation may be treated successfully by excision of the outer end of the clavicle. The recovery period is three to four weeks.

tion. Internal fixation with threaded wires is indicated when closed reduction cannot be maintained (Fig. 131).

Dislocations of the acromioclavicular articulation, even when untreated, may not cause serious disability. There may be complete dislocation, including rupture of the coracoid clavicular ligaments, without much dysfunction. When pain is present and the patient is incapacitated because of the chronic dislocation, it is advisable to repair the coracoid clavicular ligaments with fascia and at the same time secure the articulation by means of fascia lata passed through drill holes and tied securely, and reenforced for six to eight weeks with the threaded steel pins inserted as in Figure 131.

A procedure which has become increasingly popular is simple excision of the outer end of the clavicle. For acute injuries which should respond to good conservative management, a procedure that entails the loss of considerable bone substance would not appear to be justified, but for patients with old, chronic or painful dislocations, the excision of ¾ to 1 in. of the outer end of the clavicle (as described and recommended by Mumford) will restore the maximum of usefulness to the shoulder more quickly and more surely than will open operation and fascial suture (Fig. 132). The result is more satisfactory than that of arthrodesis of the acromioclavicular joint, as the latter procedure restricts shoulder motion.

Fractures of the scapula may include the body, the neck or the coracoid process. Crushing injuries, as those which result from an automobile collision or a fall from a height, may produce comminution of the blade of the scapula or a split throughout its entire length. Attempts are too often made to treat this relatively self-healing injury by immobilizing the entire arm at the patient's side. Such immobilization often produces pericapsular adhesions of the shoulder which are far more difficult to treat than the fracture itself should have been from the beginning. Little, if any, displacement occurs in this injury, and no attempt need be made to change the position of the fragments. Adhesive strapping across the shoulder and down over the back of the scapula to the level of the patient's waist will furnish all the immobilization that is needed.

A *fracture of the neck* of the scapula is much more serious than a fracture of the body. In this injury, the glenoid fossa is detached from the body of the scapula, so that the support of the arm is lost. Fortunately, the glenoid fragment can be readily controlled by manipulation or fixation of the arm, and nonunion is uncommon. In the adolescent or young adult, immobilization should be by means of an abduction arm and body cast for six weeks. The top of the arm and shoulder portion of the cast should be removed within three weeks and exercises of the arm should be started. Continuous traction may occasionally be necessary for reduction and maintenance of position. For the older patient, slight malunion is preferable to the potential danger of immobilization, namely, a frozen shoulder. A Velpeau dressing is applied for seven days or until the acute traumatic reaction has subsided. Relaxed motion is then started, with six or eight exercise periods daily. The arm is swung at the shoulder in gradually increasing circles while the patient bends forward and to the side. This will be helpful in maintaining shoulder mobility and in improving the position of the fragments. A sling attached to the wrist and passed around the neck may be worn during the intervals between the exercise periods for approximately two weeks.

A *fracture of the coracoid process* will usually repair without specific treatment, either by fibrous tissue or by solid bony union. If it occurs as a solitary lesion due to direct violence against the coracoid, no specific treatment is necessary. If the fracture is associated with a dislocation of the acromioclavicular joint, it may be treated in conjunction with, but always secondary to, the management of the acromioclavicular injury. The acromion process may be excised if it interferes with the function of the shoulder.

PART III

Fractures and Dislocations
of the Lower Limbs

CHAPTER XXIV

The Hip

THE hip is a strong and stable joint. Because of its importance in locomotion, any injury to it requires special care to assure return of satisfactory function.

TRAUMATIC DISLOCATION

Traumatic dislocation of the hip constitutes a major injury which is rarely produced by the ordinary falls that cause most fractures in this location. There are three main types, depending on the direction of displacement of the femur in relation to the acetabulum:

1. Posterior
   a) Iliac—femoral head displaced along lateral surface of iliac bone.
   b) Ischial—femoral head lies in region of sciatic notch.
2. Anterior
   a) Obturator—femoral head lies on obturator membrane.
   b) Pubic—femoral head lies external to superior ramus of pubic bone.
3. Central—femoral head displaced through acetabulum into pelvis.

The most common cause of *posterior dislocation* of the hip is that of a head-on collision of fast-moving motor cars. When the passenger's knee strikes the dashboard with the thigh in flexion and adduction, the head of the femur may be driven backward out of the acetabulum. The posterior rim of the acetabulum may be fractured at the same time. The diagnosis is seldom difficult to make from the history of a severe injury with a characteristic deformity. The involved leg appears shortened and is held in moderate hip flexion, adduction and internal rotation with the knee resting on the well leg (Fig. 133). Any attempt to move the extremity is associated with severe pain and muscle spasm. This position of the leg should not be confused with that seen after fracture of the neck of the femur with separation of the fragments, as in the latter instance the extremity is held in extension and external rotation.

Reduction of a posterior dislocation of the hip requires complete muscle relaxation, and this is obtained best by a general anesthetic. We prefer Pentothal sodium. The classic maneuver of Bigelow, illustrated in Figure 134, will rarely fail to result in re-position of the head of the femur.

Downward traction on the flexed thigh and knee with the patient lying face down and the involved leg projecting beyond the end of the table is an alternative method which may be employed for reduction. Ischial dislocations are treated the same as the iliac type. Care should be exercised to prevent injury to the sciatic nerve which occasionally becomes caught anterior to the neck of the femur and prevents closed reduction. The physician should test the function of this nerve before and following manipulative treatment of posterior dislocations of the hip.

Anterior dislocations of the hip follow severe blows to the leg with the extremity in abduction. The obturator type is the most common; the pubic dislocation represents a greater degree of upward and anterior displacement of the femur. The leg assumes a characteristic position of hip flexion, abduction and external

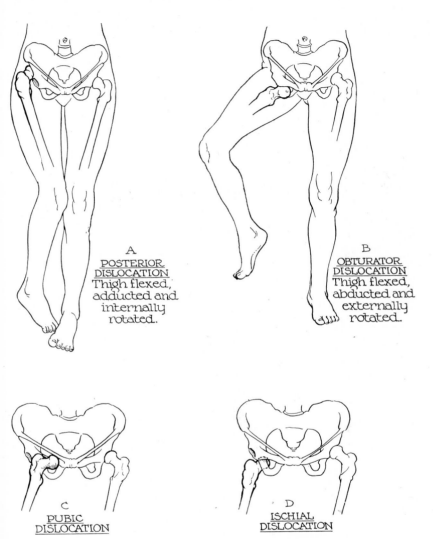

A
<u>POSTERIOR
DISLOCATION</u>
Thigh flexed,
adducted and
internally
rotated.

B
<u>OBTURATOR
DISLOCATION</u>
Thigh flexed,
abducted and
externally
rotated.

C
<u>PUBIC
DISLOCATION</u>

D
<u>ISCHIAL
DISLOCATION</u>

FIG. 133.—Four types of dislocation of the hip.

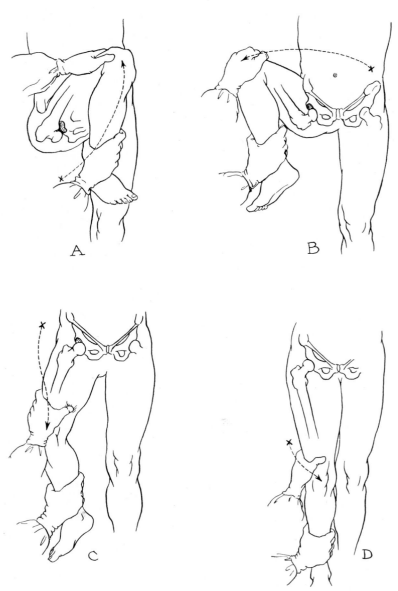

FIG. 134.—Reduction of dislocation of the hip.

rotation. Reduction may be accomplished by a reverse Bigelow maneuver, in which the flexed hip with upward traction is circumducted in a clockwise direction to a neutral position of extension. A loud click will be heard as the head pops back to position in the acetabulum.

Central dislocations of the hip are discussed in Chapter XXXI.

POST-REDUCTION TREATMENT OF TRAUMATIC DISLOCATIONS OF THE HIP

Following reduction of a posterior or anterior dislocation of the hip, the leg should be immobilized in traction with Buck's extension on a Thomas splint. Six to 8 lb. of traction is adequate to prevent re-dislocation, and a plaster cast is not necessary. Active motion of the hip and knee may be resumed after four weeks. Six weeks following the injury, the patient may become ambulatory, using crutches. The physician cannot then determine by physical examination or by roentgenograms whether the femoral head has maintained blood supply adequate for survival (see Chapter XIV), so weight-bearing on the leg should not be permitted for six months. During this period there will occur sufficient atrophy of living bone to enable the surgeon to determine by study of roentgenograms whether or not the femoral head is alive or necrotic. If the head undergoes uniform atrophy of disuse it is viable. On the other hand, if the roentgenograms show that the femoral head has retained its original density or is mottled in appearance and stands out in contrast to the less dense surrounding atrophic living bone of trochanter and pelvis, the head is necrotic. If the head is dead, two tibial bone grafts may be inserted through the neck into the head to facilitate its restitution (Fig. 32). The patient should continue to use crutches for walking without bearing weight on the affected leg, until there is roentgenographic evidence of complete transformation of the femoral head. Transformation of the head may require several years, but the treatment is worth while if a deformed and painful joint requiring osteotomy, arthroplasty or arthrodesis of the hip can be prevented.

When this program is not followed and the patient is permitted to resume walking six weeks after the dislocation, he may have normal function of the hip for six to 10 months even though the head has lost its blood supply. Too frequently these

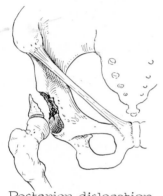

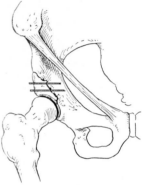

Posterior dislocation
of hip with fracture
of the acetabulum

Dislocation reduced
and fragment wired
in place with threaded
wires

Fig. 135.—Open operation for accurate reduction and fixation of all large acetabular fragments is recommended.

patients will return to the physician with pain and spasm around the hip and roentgenograms will show late evidence of necrosis with variable degrees of breakdown of the head.

Complications of dislocations of the hip are: (1) aseptic necrosis of the femoral head from tearing of major blood vessels at the time of the injury; (2) displacement of large acetabular fragments which may require open reduction and internal fixation (Figs. 135 and 136); (3) myositis ossificans and ossification of the capsule which occasionally cause marked loss of motion in the hip joint; (4) injury to the sciatic nerve.

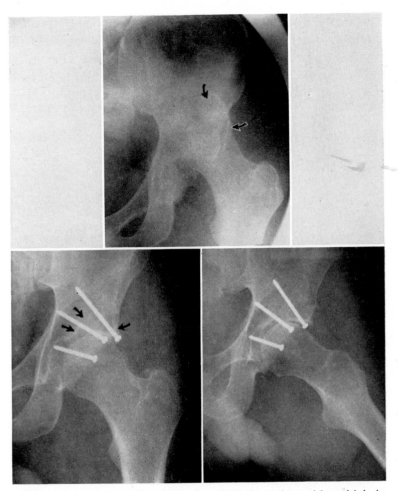

Fig. 136.—Severe fracture dislocation of hip in patient with multiple injuries incurred when he jumped from a burning airplane just before it crashed. Large fragment representing about one third of the acetabulum (indicated by arrows) was accurately replaced with three screws. Eighteen months after injury roentgenograms demonstrate an apparently viable head with moderate narrowing of the joint space. Full weight-bearing had been permitted for six months.

The most frequent severe complication is aseptic necrosis. The incidence is high (probably 40 per cent of all cases), and the crippling end-result may produce marked disability (Fig. 137).

Old unreduced dislocations of the hip offer little hope for a good result. Rarely can closed reduction be accomplished three

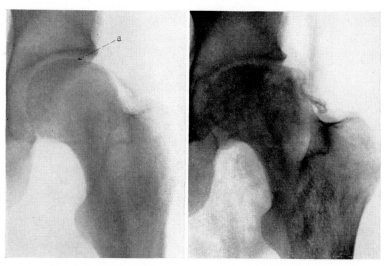

Fig. 137.—*Left,* roentgenogram of hip of man, aged 24, 13 months after closed reduction of a posterior dislocation. Recurrence of pain after eight months of normal function and minimal flattening of the head (*a*) indicate vascular deficiency of the head. Note the lack of contrast density. *Right,* 43 months after dislocation and 34 months after return of pain. Hip was protected by crutches with restitution of head, but this did not prevent flattening of the weight-bearing surface and marginal proliferation of bone.

weeks after the dislocation, and open reduction will be followed by necrosis of the femoral head in most instances. If the femoral head can be replaced in the acetabulum, arthrodesis offers the most favorable prognosis for a stable, painless weight-bearing extremity. Arthroplasty has also been advised, but after this operation a necrotic femoral head may collapse and be absorbed beneath the vitallium cup. A subtrochanteric osteotomy is advisable for unreducible dislocations of the hip, with displacement of the femoral shaft medially to improve stability.

FRACTURES

Fractures in the region of the hip should be divided into two major groups: (1) fractures that occur within the capsule of the joint, and (2) those which occur at the base of the neck with involvement of one or both trochanters. The prognosis for union and restoration of normal function varies considerably in the two groups.

The blood supply of the femoral head is derived from the nutrient branches of the anterior and posterior circumflex arteries which enter the epiphysis after passing beneath the reflection of the capsule on the neck of the femur and from the arteries of the round ligament (Figs. 138 and 139). The capsular vessels are more important than are those of the ligamentum teres. In intracapsular fractures with displacement, the neck vessels will be torn. The blood supply through the round ligament may not be sufficient to nourish the entire femoral head and aseptic necrosis will inevitably result unless some of the capsular vessels remain intact. Basal neck and intertrochanteric fractures occur distal to the hip joint capsule and rarely sever important arteries.

The acute slipped epiphysis or epiphyseal line fracture, which occurs in adolescents, takes place within the capsule and may leave only the blood supply available by way of the round ligament. The vessels in the round ligament are of larger caliber in children than in adults, and comparable fractures in young individuals carry a more favorable prognosis. Gradual slipping of the femoral epiphysis probably permits readjustment of the blood supply by the capsular vessels and together with the supply through the ligamentum teres no doubt accounts for the low incidence of or delayed necrosis which results from this lesion.

SLIPPING OF THE FEMORAL EPIPHYSIS in adolescents should be recognized early, before any marked displacement has occurred. It can be treated successfully by wide abduction and

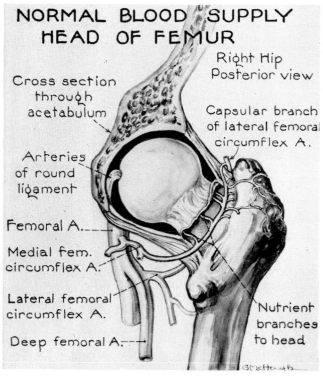

NORMAL BLOOD SUPPLY
HEAD OF FEMUR

Cross section
through
acetabulum

Right Hip
Posterior view

Capsular branch
of lateral femoral
circumflex A.

Arteries
of round
ligament

Femoral A.

Medial fem.
circumflex A.

Lateral femoral
circumflex A.

Deep femoral A.

Nutrient
branches
to head

FIG. 138.

internal rotation in a plaster cast for four to six months. We prefer internal fixation with threaded steel pins or a Smith-Petersen nail because this does not require immobilization of an entire extremity and therefore permits ambulation with crutches without weight-bearing on the affected hip. The procedure for insertion of the pins or nail is that outlined for intracapsular fractures of the hip (Figs. 146 and 144). Weight-bearing may be resumed when roentgenograms show bony fusion between the head and the neck. Late development of pain with roentgen evidence of altered contour of the head suggests the possibility

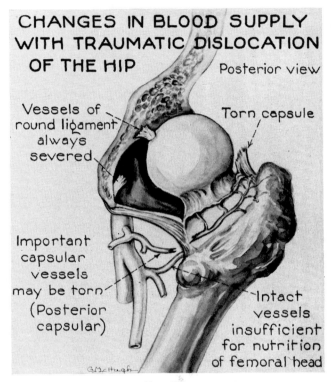

CHANGES IN BLOOD SUPPLY WITH TRAUMATIC DISLOCATION OF THE HIP   Posterior view

Vessels of round ligament always severed

Torn capsule

Important capsular vessels may be torn (Posterior capsular)

Intact vessels insufficient for nutrition of femoral head

FIG. 139.

of aseptic necrosis, and the patient should be treated accordingly by prolonged protection against weight-bearing.

TRUE FRACTURES OF THE FEMORAL NECK.—These are common among elderly individuals, since they are more susceptible to falls, such as tripping on a rug or slipping in a bath tub. Frequently the injury results from a fall in which the patient strikes the side of the hip. Impaction of the fracture fragments may enable the patient to walk without great difficulty (Fig. 140). However, unless the fracture is recognized and adequately

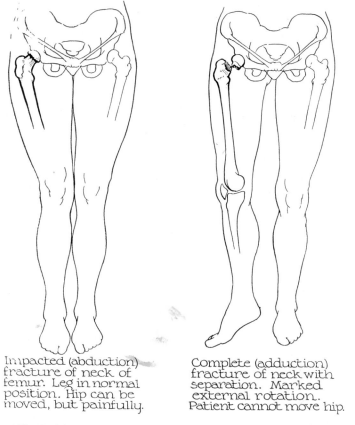

Impacted (abduction) fracture of neck of femur. Leg in normal position. Hip can be moved, but painfully.

Complete (adduction) fracture of neck with separation. Marked external rotation. Patient cannot move hip.

FIG. 140.—Position of the leg following intracapsular fractures of the hip.

treated within a few days, displacement, with a poor prognosis, may follow. Because so many of these patients are elderly, the incidence of death from hypostatic pneumonia or from cardio-renal failure was high with cast treatment but has been mate-

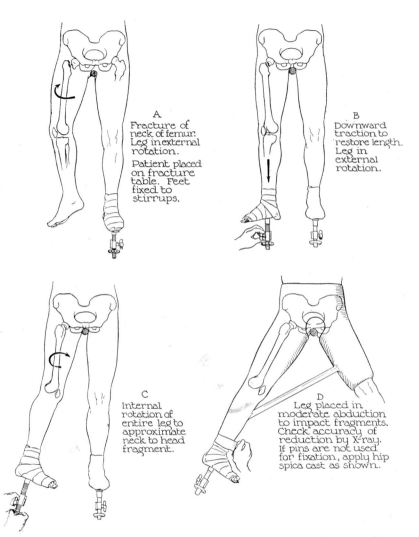

A
Fracture of neck of femur. Leg in external rotation.

Patient placed on fracture table. Feet fixed to stirrups.

B
Downward traction to restore length. Leg in external rotation.

C
Internal rotation of entire leg to approximate neck to head fragment.

D
Leg placed in moderate abduction to impact fragments. Check accuracy of reduction by X-ray. If pins are not used for fixation, apply hip spica cast as shown.

FIG. 141.—Whitman method of treatment for intracapsular fracture of the hip. While the authors utilize this method for reduction, they recommend internal fixation in preference to the plaster spica cast for immobilization.

269

rially reduced by early ambulation after internal fixation of the fracture.

No attempt at reduction should be made while there is any evidence of shock. During the first 24 hours after admission, Buck's extension may be applied to the leg and the extremity gradually rotated to a neutral position and supported with sandbags. The head of the bed should be kept elevated and the patient turned at frequent intervals, in an effort to prevent hypostatic congestion of the lungs.

Use of the plaster cast has been abandoned by men who know the discipline required for good fracture therapy (Fig. 141). The prognosis for a good functional result with bone union is fully twice as good when internal fixation is skilfully applied following an accurate reduction. Furthermore, the patient is much more comfortable and happy during the course of treatment, and is far more likely to survive it, if he is able to sit up, to ride in a wheel chair or, when not too feeble, to use crutches and walk, without weight-bearing on the leg in which the fracture is being treated.

In the elderly patient, it may be advisable to avoid any type of regional or general anesthetic. Sufficient relaxation to reduce and immobilize the fracture internally may be secured by local infiltration of 1 per cent procaine, preceded one hour by 1/150 gr. of scopolamine and one-half hour by 1/4 gr. of morphine. The procaine should be injected directly into the hematoma at the site of fracture and also infiltrated into the skin over the lateral surface of the femur below the greater trochanter. The use of alcohol intravenously as described in Chapter V is especially indicated for the poor risk, elderly patient.

In obtaining reduction, the surgeon should strive to produce both accurate apposition of the fracture surfaces and a definite coxa valga position; nothing short of this should be considered satisfactory. Most failures, and no doubt some aseptic necroses of femoral heads, can be attributed to inadequate reduction or failure to obtain complete immobilization by whatever method of internal fixation is employed. Pauwels, more than anyone else, should be given credit for emphasizing the need of relieving the shearing stress, which is produced by muscle pull and weight-bearing, on the line of fracture of the neck of the femur. The more horizontal the fracture line, the less this strain. The more vertical the fracture line, the more difficult it is to maintain perfect apposition of the fracture fragments and to prevent slipping in the line of fracture. Fractures with early union have been observed to break down after a period of weight-bearing activity, because this shearing force on a relatively perpendicular line of fracture was not relieved by obtaining a reduction in which the head of the femur was replaced more directly on top of the neck.

REDUCTION OF FEMORAL NECK FRACTURES

The method of reduction may be outlined as follows:
1. Direct downward traction in the line of the long axis of the femur and tibia.
2. Abduction of the leg, through an arc of 10 to 20 degrees, while traction is being maintained.
3. Internal rotation of the leg until the patella faces medially (Fig. 141).

This method can be most safely carried out with the patient on a fracture table with both feet firmly fastened to the traction stirrups. A wooden perineal post should be used to facilitate the taking of check-up roentgenograms. A hospital fracture service which has secured the full co-operation of the department of roentgenology will have portable equipment available for taking both anteroposterior and lateral roentgenograms of the hip. Satisfactory results in a series of fractures of the neck of the femur cannot be obtained without the aid of two-plane roentgen examinations made immediately after each manipulation to reduce the fracture, at various times during the process of internal

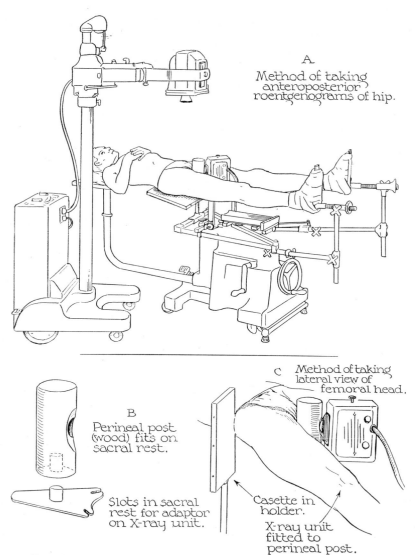

A
Method of taking anteroposterior roentgenograms of hip.

B
Perineal post (wood) fits on sacral rest.

Slots in sacral rest for adaptor on X-ray unit.

C Method of taking lateral view of femoral head.

Casette in holder.

X-ray unit fitted to perineal post.

FIG. 142.—Equipment for obtaining anteroposterior and lateral roentgenograms (Dr. Hugh McKenna, Chicago). This method may be used for repeated roentgenograms during an open operative procedure without interrupting the sterile technique.

272

fixation and as a final check-up before sending the patient back to his room.

The arrangement is ideal when two portable x-ray tubes are provided. One tube should be fastened by special brackets to the fracture table and placed between the patient's thighs, with the opening as close to the inner side of the groin as possible and directed upward toward the neck of the femur (Fig. 142). This tube is covered with sterile drapes and does not need to be disturbed when lateral roentgenograms are called for. A cassette holder for 8 × 10 film is placed beneath the hip and so arranged that it will be easy to insert and remove the x-ray cassettes as anteroposterior films are required. A portable x-ray machine can be used to take anteroposterior views.

LEADBETTER MANEUVER

Occasionally a satisfactory reduction by simple traction, abduction and internal rotation is not obtained. The Leadbetter maneuver should be used in these cases (Fig. 143). With the knee and thigh flexed a little more than 90 degrees, an upward lift on the leg is made until the pelvis is elevated. The thigh is internally circumducted and internally rotated; as the leg is extended, the internal rotation is maintained and the leg is carried laterally to a position of 35 degree abduction. The Leadbetter test (Fig. 143, *D*) may then be applied: When the leg is supported with the heel of the patient's foot resting on the palm of the surgeon's hand, the foot will not rotate externally, but will remain vertical or turned slightly into internal rotation, if reduction is satisfactory and one fracture fragment engages the other.

The anteroposterior roentgenogram of the completely reduced hip should show the head of the femur well up onto the neck, creating a definite coxa valga position, and the lesser trochanter will be almost if not entirely hidden behind the shaft of the femur. If the lesser trochanter shows in prominent profile in an anteroposterior film, the surgeon can be reasonably certain that

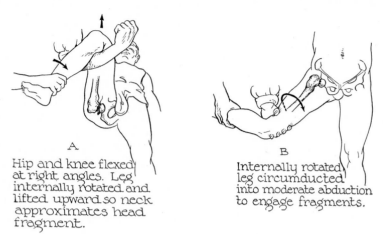

A

Hip and knee flexed
at right angles. Leg
internally rotated and
lifted upward so neck
approximates head
fragment.

B

Internally rotated
leg circumducted
into moderate abduction
to engage fragments.

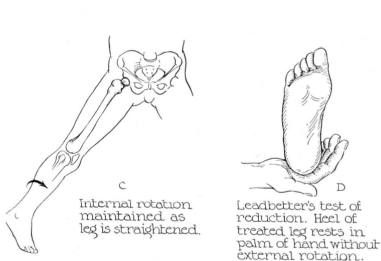

C

Internal rotation
maintained as
leg is straightened.

D

Leadbetter's test of
reduction. Heel of
treated leg rests in
palm of hand without
external rotation.

FIG. 143.—Leadbetter's method of reduction of intracapsular fracture of
the hip.

the reduction is not satisfactory and the internal rotation should be increased.

INTERNAL FIXATION OF FEMORAL NECK

For many years, we preferred and used small threaded steel pins, inserted without incision of the skin or through a lateral incision, for immobilization of fresh intracapsular fractures of the neck of the femur. These pins effectively maintained immobilization if they were accurately placed after reduction of the fracture. Difficulty in procuring the best quality of surgical steel during World War II resulted in a loss of confidence in the small threaded steel pins and the discontinuance of their use except in fractures of smaller bones and for immobilizing the reduced capital epiphysis following epiphysiolysis. The lag screw, long wood screws, partially threaded pins, angle blade plates and other materials for internal fixation of fractures of the femoral neck have been satisfactory when used by men who were well trained in the appropriate techniques. All of these methods have been used by us at one time or another. We now prefer, and use in most instances of recent fracture of the intracapsular portion of the neck of the femur, Smith-Petersen nails. It should be noted that this nail is most efficiently used when the femoral bone is not extensively atrophic. The bones of patients who have been long inactive because of far advanced years may not be strong enough to prevent the nail from coming out through the anterior cortex of the neck or through the head of the femur, or from backing out until the fracture fragments are no longer maintained in position. When dealing with bone of this type, the use of a three-flange nail and plate which can be attached to the side of the femur is desirable. With rare exceptions we use the closed method of reduction of the fracture and insert the Smith-Petersen nail through a 5 in. lateral incision. Whether or not the fracture line is exposed, roentgenographic control, with both lateral and anterior posterior films during the operation, is essential.

TECHNIQUE (MODIFICATION OF SMITH-PETERSEN, FIG. 144)

1. Place the patient on the fracture table with the uninjured leg attached to the foot piece.

2. Reduce the fracture by the Leadbetter (Fig. 143) or the Whitman (Fig. 141) method, or as described on page 271. With the leg in traction, continue sufficient pull to keep the leg just taut. Excessive pull will disengage the fragments. The leg is rotated by grasping the thigh and turning the foot piece so that the patella is directed inward. About 15 degrees of abduction will bring the head fragment into valgus and simultaneously maintain contact between the fragments. Excessive abduction may create a gap between the head and neck in the medial half of the fracture. The pelvis is balanced by applying the necessary amount of traction on the well leg.

3. Apply a Michel clip on the skin over Poupart's ligament midway between the anterior superior iliac spine and pubic tubercle. This clip should be identified on the roentgenograms and is the target toward which the guide pin will be directed.

4. Check reduction by anteroposterior and lateral roentgenograms of the hip. Two portable roentgen units are indispensable for roentgenographing quickly and without disturbing the sterile drapes (Fig. 142).

5. Scrub the skin for 10 minutes from the ribs to the knee with soap containing a detergent. Apply an antiseptic.

6. Re-position the fracture if roentgenograms do not show an adequate reduction. The fracture is properly reduced when the head is in a position of valgus with good contact with the neck and when the lesser trochanter cannot be seen. The skin clip marker is placed over the midpoint of Poupart's ligament and the surgical field is properly draped.

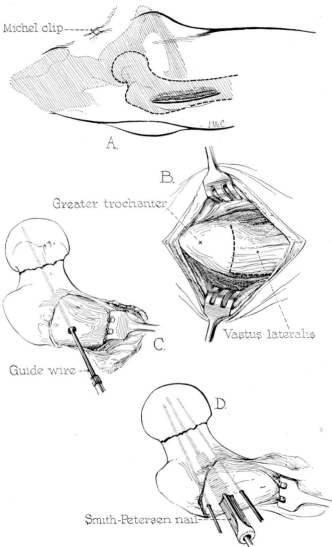

Fig. 144.—Introduction of a Smith-Petersen nail for internal fixation of intracapsular fractures of the neck of the femur.

7. The skin incision begins over the lateral tip of the greater trochanter and extends downward 5 in. Incise the fascia lata. Raise the periosteum and vastus lateralis from the subtrochanteric portion of the femur. Detach the muscle at the base of the trochanter for additional exposure.

8. Place two ¼ in. drill holes in the lateral cortex of the femur 1–1½ in. distal to the base of the greater trochanter. They should be ½ in. apart and directed toward the Michel clip which marks on the skin the approximate location of the head of the femur.

9. Pass a Smith-Petersen nail guide wire (do not substitute a Kirschner wire) through each hole into the neck and head of the femur. One should enter the bone for 4 in. and the other 3¾ in. to permit roentgenographic identification and to give information as to the length of nail required. The wires are inserted parallel to the floor (if the extremity is in proper degree of internal rotation) and aimed in the direction of the clip marker. The wires are pushed in (without drilling) until increased resistance is encountered, indicating that the head fragment has been reached. The wires are drilled into the head, one not quite as deep as the other.

10. Determine the position of the wires by anteroposterior and lateral roentgenograms. Readjust the length and position of the wires if one is not located in the center of the neck and head. Re-check their location roentgenographically. The wires are re-inserted one at a time, using the other one in the bone as a guide for the new direction. Repeat the adjustment of the wires until the position of one wire is perfect. Do not insert the Smith-Petersen nail until a guide wire is in the ideal position. *An inadequate nailing is doomed to failure.*

11. Select a Smith-Petersen nail of proper length by subtracting the length of guide wire protruding from the femur

from the total length of the wire. The difference represents the length of the wire inside the bone, and this length on the anteroposterior roentgenogram is used for accurate determination of the required length of nail.

12. Prepare the femoral cortex at the point where the guide pin is inserted to accept the three blades of the nail. A Smith-Petersen nail starter, a cannulated burr designed for this purpose or a small osteotome may be used.

13. Insert the Smith-Petersen nail into the femoral neck over the guide pin. Hold the nail in line with the wire, with the attached cannulated nail holder, to prevent bending the guide pin. Remove the second guide wire if its position interferes with the insertion of the nail; otherwise, it may be left in place to minimize the danger of rotation of the head fragment as the nail is inserted. Remove the guide wires and check by roentgenogram the position and depth to which the nail has been inserted. Do not transfix the end of the nail to the lateral cortex of the femur. The nail should be free to back out of the femur as impaction takes place, either with or without absorption of the bone at the fracture site.

14. The fragments are impacted with the Smith-Petersen impactor and the wound is closed. Apply a local pressure dressing, using Elastoplast part way around the leg.

15. The patient is returned to bed with 5 lb. of traction applied by means of adhesive strips or a threaded pin through the proximal end of the tibia. This minimizes muscle spasm and controls the position of the extremity (prevents sudden external rotary movements which may disengage the fragments) until active motion is possible.

16. An elderly patient should be up in a wheel chair each day, while more vigorous persons are kept in bed until muscle spasm has disappeared. This usually requires five to seven days.

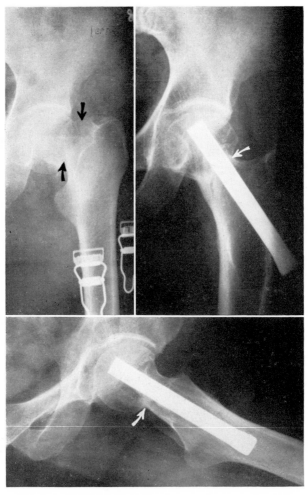

Fɪɢ. 145.—Subcapital fracture of the neck of the femur treated by slight overcorrection into a valgus position and internal fixation with a Smith-Petersen nail.

17. Repeat roentgen examination 10 to 14 days after surgery at which time the femur can be flexed 90 degrees for the lateral view (Fig. 145). For the anteroposterior roentgenogram, the extremity must be rotated internally so that the entire neck containing the nail can be seen in profile.

18. Physically able patients may be discharged from the hospital soon thereafter, walking on the good leg with the help of crutches. Crutch walking is assisted by build-up of the heel of the shoe about ½ in. on the uninjured extremity.

19. Weight-bearing is allowed when anteroposterior and lateral roentgenograms show obliteration of the fracture line by bone. Rarely does callus form on the surface of the femoral neck, union occurring by intramedullary bone formation instead. Fractures of the neck of the femur usually require 4½ to six months to heal, but occasionally union takes place in three to 3½ months. Consolidation may be delayed for many months as a result of poor reduction, ineffective nail insertion or aseptic necrosis of the femoral head.

20. The nail is not removed routinely unless it has entered the hip joint, has cut out of the neck into the surrounding soft tissues or unless a painful bursa has formed over the end that protrudes laterally from the shaft of the femur. Removal of the nail is delayed, unless circumstances dictate otherwise, until union takes place.

For those who prefer to use the threaded stainless steel pins, we submit the following description of the technique which we have used (Fig. 146). The pins may be inserted directly through the skin and into the bone by a cannulated Yankee drill. The landmarks which were originally described for insertion of the Moore nails are used as guides for insertion of the pins. They are started as nearly as possible at the four angles of a quadrant

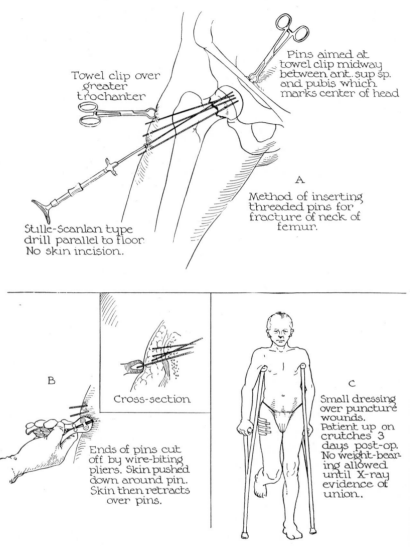

Towel clip over greater trochanter

Pins aimed at towel clip midway between ant. sup sp. and pubis which marks center of head

A

Method of inserting threaded pins for fracture of neck of femur.

Stille-Scanlan type drill parallel to floor. No skin incision.

B

Cross-section

C

Small dressing over puncture wounds. Patient up on crutches 3 days post-op. No weight-bearing allowed until X-ray evidence of union.

Ends of pins cut off by wire-biting pliers. Skin pushed down around pin. Skin then retracts over pins.

Fig. 146.—Internal fixation of a recent fracture of the neck of the femur by small threaded pins.

which may be drawn on the skin with iodine or gentian violet at a level 1½ in. below the tip of the greater trochanter. The drill and pin are held parallel to the level of the top of the fracture table, centered against the side of the femur, and are directed, as one would aim a gun, at a point indicated by a clip on the skin halfway between the anterior superior spine of the ilium and the pubic bone. After inserting two pins to a depth previously determined by measurements on the roentgenograms, usually about 3½ in., anteroposterior and lateral roentgenograms are again made. The pins should be found to stay well within the substance of the neck and to enter the head of the femur. If the roentgenographic check-up shows that the pins are correctly placed, two additional pins are inserted. If not properly centered they should be removed and replaced.

Ideally, the pins are inserted so that one is anterior, posterior, superior and inferior in the quadrants of the femoral neck. They should be adjusted for depth by drilling them slightly forward, or withdrawing them, as may be indicated by studying the roentgenograms. The points of the pins should not reach the cortex of the articular surface of the head. Atrophy and absorption at the line of fracture will invariably produce some shortening of the neck, and if the points of the pins reach too close to the cortex of the head, they later may protrude through and into the joint as the absorption takes place.

When final roentgenograms have been made and the positions of the immobilizing threaded pins have been found to be entirely satisfactory, the skin is depressed inward toward the trochanter as far as possible, and each pin is cut off with a heavy nipper. The skin is then permitted to retract outward, leaving the ends of the pins buried at a depth of 1½ to 2 in. in obese patients and ½ to 1 in. in others. The ends of the pins cause only slight discomfort. If the patient complains of them later, they can be removed, but not less than six months after reduction of the fracture.

A patient who has been treated by this method requires no plaster cast and no other form of external immobilization. He may be permitted to sit up in bed or in a wheel chair on the afternoon following operation. Within two or three days, a patient so treated may walk with crutches, assisted by two nurses or other attendants, if he is strong enough to support his weight on the well leg, and within a week or two he should be able to leave the hospital. Internal fixation techniques have greatly reduced the cost of hospital care for fractures of the neck of the femur. The immediate activity which they permit is undoubtedly an important factor in the physiologic recovery. Weight-bearing is not permitted until solid union is demonstrated roentgenographically. This usually requires six months.

NONUNION OF FRACTURES of the neck of the femur is usually the result of poor reduction or inadequate immobilization of the fracture. Frequently, it is the result of aseptic necrosis of the head (see Chapter XIV). Many methods have been described for treating nonunion of this fracture (Figs. 147 and 148). These vary from extensive reconstruction operations, some utilizing the femoral head (Magnuson and Brackett), to those in which the head is removed entirely and the trochanter deflected laterally or transplanted downward onto the shaft. They are briefly described for the purpose of familiarizing the general practitioner or student with possible procedures. The execution of each procedure requires special skill and experience, and a detailed presentation of each method is not within the scope of this book.

The result to be hoped for is restoration, as nearly as possible, of a normal anatomic relationship and good physiologic function. Good results have been reported from the use of tibial bone grafts (Fig. 149). Our original objection to this method has been that it required long immobilization in a body and leg plaster cast of a patient who in all probability had already been subjected to an extensive period of physical inactivity in the

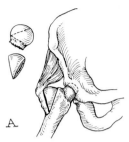

A

Wedge made from removed
head of femur and fitted into
split trochanter.   Neck of
femur reduced into acetabulum.
(Albee)

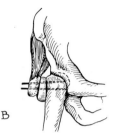

B

Trochanter reduced into
acetabulum. Portions of
head and trochanter pinned
to shaft.
(Campbell)

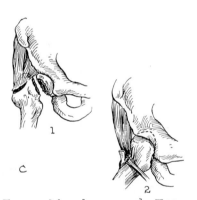

C

Femoral head removed. Trochanter reduced into acetabulum.
Abductor muscles transplanted
down on shaft.
(Colonna)

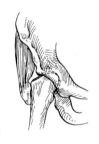

D

Head of femur removed. Neck
reduced into acetabulum.
Trochanter with abductor
muscles displaced down on shaft.
(Whitman)

Fig. 147.—Operations that have been recommended for treatment of old
ununited fractures of the hip with necrosis of the femoral head.

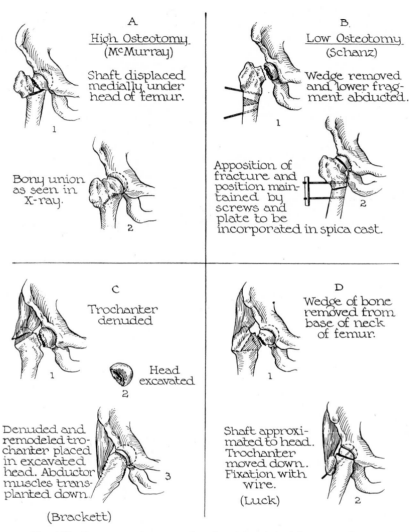

A
High Osteotomy.
(McMurray)

Shaft displaced
medially under
head of femur.

1

Bony union
as seen in
X-ray.

2

B.
Low Osteotomy.
(Schanz)

Wedge removed
and lower frag-
ment abducted.

1

Apposition of
fracture and
position main-
tained by
screws and
plate to be
incorporated in spica cast.

2

C
Trochanter
denuded

1

Head
excavated

2

Denuded and
remodeled tro-
chanter placed
in excavated
head. Abductor
muscles trans-
planted down.

3

(Brackett)

D
Wedge of bone
removed from
base of neck
of femur.

1

Shaft approxi-
mated to head.
Trochanter
moved down.
Fixation with
wire.

(Luck)

2

FIG. 148.—Reconstruction operations for old ununited fractures of the neck
of the femur with viable femoral heads. The use of a blade plate or a Smith-
Petersen nail with a plate attachment might preclude the use of a hip spica
cast.

treatment of the fresh fracture. This attitude has been modified as follows.

We have used, in chosen cases with roentgenographic evidence of a viable head, an operation for open reduction of the fracture

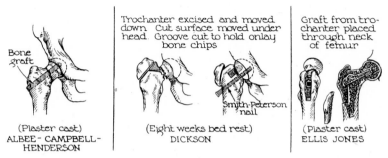

FIG. 149.—Other techniques in which a bone graft has been used to aid in obtaining osteosynthesis in ununited fractures of the hip.

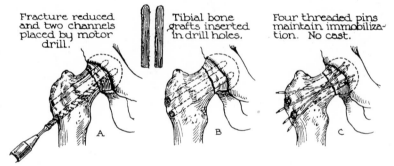

FIG. 150.—Method of treatment of nonunion of fractures of the hip used by the authors if the femoral head is viable. It permits early ambulation.

fragments to obtain a position of accurate apposition and slight valgus (Fig. 150). Two autogenous tibial bone grafts are inserted laterally from below the greater trochanter up through the neck and into the head fragment. Four threaded steel pins are then used to give support and maintain immobilization while union is taking place, stimulated by the autogenous and osteogenetic effect of the bone grafts (Fig. 151). No cast is needed (unless the bone is too osteoporotic for the pins to maintain the reduction), and postoperative hospitalization may be reduced to three weeks.

Subtrochanteric osteotomy, of the types recommended by

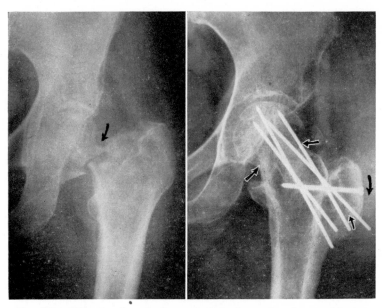

Fig. 151.—Old nonunion of a fracture of the femoral neck treated by intra-medullary autogenous bone grafts with threaded wire fixation. The greater trochanter was transplanted downward and fixed with a stainless steel screw. The roentgenogram shows uniform atrophy of the head of the femur and this was interpreted as being indicative of a live head. This procedure should not be used when necrosis of the femoral head is obvious at the time of operation.

McMurray and by Schanz, is a procedure which produces ex-cellent results (Fig. 148, *A* and *B*). The McMurray type of osteotomy is recommended because the technique is relatively simple and the end-results are highly satisfactory. Either type of osteotomy requires an additional period of plaster cast immobili-zation of 8 to 12 weeks unless some form of internal fixation is used. A combination flange and plate holds the bones, after osteotomy and abduction or medial displacement of the distal fragment, without requiring immobilization of the extremity in a plaster cast.

Nonunion, with or without a viable head, occurring in the very elderly patient constitutes an indication for use of a plastic or metallic replacement. We formerly used the reinforced acrylic prosthesis modified from Judet, but now use, with much improved results, the Eicher stainless steel prosthesis. The posterior lateral incision, described by Gibson, provides an excellent exposure of the hip joint. The incision begins at the posterior superior spine of the ilium, is carried laterally toward the tip of the greater trochanter and down along the shaft of the femur for a distance of 5 or 6 in. The gluteus maximus muscle is retracted medially, and the gluteus medius muscle laterally. The abductor muscles are detached from the trochanter and reflected proximally to expose the joint capsule. The necrotic head of the femur is removed. The prosthesis is inserted with the stem placed through the base of the femoral neck and down the shaft in a channel previously prepared with a broach or drill. Traction for three to seven days, with the leg abducted 15 degrees and internally rotated slightly, is sufficient immobilization. Early ambulation in a walker or with crutches, while weight-bearing is encouraged, is recommended.

INTERTROCHANTERIC FRACTURES.—All fractures of the hip which are outside the joint capsule have been grouped under the general heading of basal neck and intertrochanteric fractures. Fractures which involve the intertrochanteric region may be oblique along the intertrochanteric line or extremely comminuted, involving fragments of both trochanters and the proximal end of the shaft of the femur. These fractures are produced by direct trauma. They may occur to an occupant of an automobile which is struck from the side by a rapidly moving car, but most often the injury is produced by a fall in the home or on a sidewalk. This injury is more common in men than in women, whereas the reverse is true of intracapsular fracture of the neck of the femur. The bone in the region of the greater trochanters is predominantly cancellous and possesses a rich supply of blood from many nutrient arteries. Nonunion of fractures in this region is exceedingly rare. Malunion with coxa vara deformity, however, occurs very frequently.

MANAGEMENT

The simplest method of treatment consists of continuous Russell traction, with a pin placed through the proximal fourth of the tibia. Buck's adhesive extension applied to the skin from the lower third of the thigh downward can be used, but this requires careful daily supervision to prevent embarrassment of the circulation, dermatitis from the adhesive and to see that the traction does not slip off. Traction must be continued for approximately 12 weeks. The weight applied to the traction must be sufficient to reduce the fracture completely and to create a few degrees of coxa valga. If traction is discontinued or weight is borne before the roentgenograms demonstrate solid union, coxa vara with shortening and a permanently weak hip may result.

For elderly patients who do not tolerate prolonged bed rest, and for younger patients in economic circumstances not permitting prolonged hospitalization, we prefer open operation with internal fixation by means of a Smith-Petersen nail with a plate extension or a flange with plate attached (Fig. 152).

The patient is placed on the fracture table with both lower extremities in strong traction. If the fracture is at the base of the femoral neck, the injured leg is internally rotated and abducted 15 degrees. In intertrochanteric fractures, the leg is placed in a neutral position or one of moderate external rotation, depending on the degree of rotation of the proximal fragment. Anteroposterior and lateral roentgenograms are then taken in order that the accuracy of the final reduction may be confirmed.

The proximal 5 in. of the subtrochanteric portion of the femur is exposed through a lateral incision. Guide wires are inserted as described for the introduction of a Smith-Petersen nail in the treatment of an intracapsular fracture of the femoral neck (Fig. 144). A Smith-Petersen nail is inserted over the guide wire so that it traverses the center of the neck and ends deep in the head.

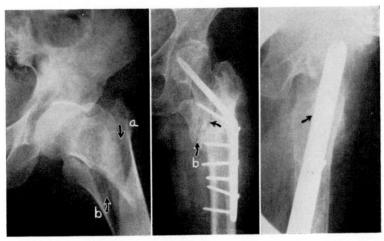

Fig. 152.—Typical comminuted intertrochanteric fracture, *a,* with separation of the lesser trochanter, *b.* Treated satisfactorily with a blade plate and no external immobilization. A three-flange nail with solid or separate plate is now our preferred method of treating these fractures.

A plate is attached to the end of the nail by a bolt or two nuts and to the lateral aspect of the femoral shaft by multiple screws. Parham bands may be used for additional stability when severe comminution is present (Fig. 11). After closure of the wound and application of a local pressure dressing, the patient is returned to bed and adhesive or skeletal traction is resumed. If the bone is atrophic, or if there is severe comminution, it may be necessary to continue traction for three to six weeks in order to avoid re-displacement of the fracture. If the fracture is stable,

the patient may become ambulatory with crutches, without
weight-bearing on the involved leg. He can then be discharged
from the hospital as soon thereafter as circumstances permit.

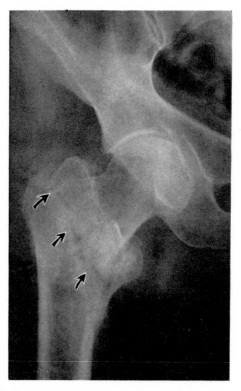

Fig. 153.—End-result of a displaced intertrochanteric fracture treated by
the well-leg traction cast method. If open reduction is contraindicated because
of the patient's condition or the extreme comminution of the proximal third
of the femur, well-leg traction may be the method of choice.

The operative procedure will vary slightly when a one-piece
flange, a plate with multiple screws or threaded wires or other
types of devices are used for internal fixation. We prefer the
Smith-Petersen nail and separate plate because it is less difficult

to insert the nail into the head when it is not permanently attached to the plate. This is especially true when the head fragment is in marked external rotation. The results from internal fixation of intertrochanteric fractures will be satisfactory in a high percentage of cases regardless of the type of device used for fixation, provided the patients are carefully selected and the procedure is properly performed.

The well-leg traction splint has proved satisfactory for reducing and maintaining good position of basal neck and intertrochanteric fractures when the patient's condition or special circumstances prohibit open reduction (Fig. 153). Steinmann pins are drilled through the supramalleolar portions of both tibiae and long leg casts are applied. After the plaster has set, the ends of the pins are placed through holes in the metal stirrups of the well-leg traction splint and the stirrups are attached to the casts by additional rolls of plaster. The fractured leg is kept in a neutral or externally rotated position, depending on the degree of external rotation of the proximal fragment.

The patient can be turned face down in bed or allowed up in a wheel chair without loss of reduction. The splint is removed after union of the fracture has taken place. This requires six to 12 weeks or more.

The well-leg traction splint is safe and effective when Steinmann pins are placed through both tibiae. Downward traction on the injured side is obtained by creating an equal pressure upward on the other leg. If this pressure is exerted on the soft tissues of the plantar aspect of the foot instead of on a Steinmann pin through the tibia, a large slough will result. *Do not apply the well-leg traction splint unless Steinmann pins are used in both tibiae.*

Dr. A. A. Mertz of Decatur, Ill., has described a method for treating intertrochanteric fractures by means of two pins placed through the distal third of the femur and the application of a bilateral short hip spica cast. The method consists of reduction of the fracture by traction and slight internal rotation. Two Steinmann pins or heavy threaded steel wires are then inserted through the femur just above the knee on the side of the frac-

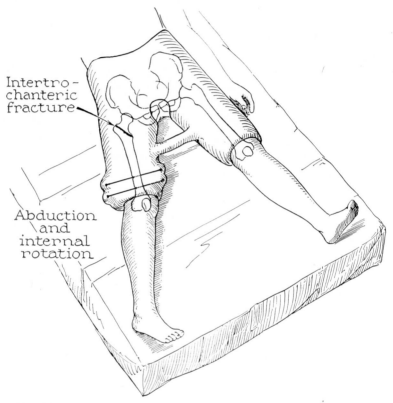

Intertro-
chanteric
fracture

Abduction
and
internal
rotation

Fig. 154.—The pantaloon cast incorporating the ends of two Steinmann pins which transfix the femur permits knee joint motion. Described by Dr. A. A. Mertz, Decatur, Ill.

ture. A "pantaloon" cast is applied (Fig. 154). The term "pantaloon" describes well the short spica cast which extends from about the level of the crests of the ilii downward. The ends of the pins are incorporated in the cast, which does not reach to the knee, permitting free exercise of the knee joints. A heavy stick is attached by plaster across the thighs, both anteriorly and posteriorly. By using this method or the well-leg traction splint, it is possible to send the patient home from the hospital within two or three days after the injury. Nursing care can be administered by other members of the family, who are instructed in the need of turning the patient several times each day and getting him up in a chair. We consider these methods less suited for the elderly patient than that of internal fixation which may permit ambulation with crutches throughout the course of healing. The methods are not technically difficult and are far more efficient and less conducive to atrophy and loss of joint function than is the long spica cast of Whitman. They are preferred also to the Russell traction method, because they permit much greater activity by the patient and do not require prolonged hospitalization.

CHAPTER XXV

The Femur

FRACTURES of the shaft of the femur occur most often in men, and during the most active period of life. Industrial accidents, falls from window ledges or scaffoldings, and automobile accidents are responsible for the majority of these injuries, which may result in transverse, oblique or torsion fractures (Fig. 155). When the break is produced by severe direct violence, there may be extreme comminution.

Because the femur is contained within an envelope of large muscles which are richly supplied with arteries and the bone itself is highly vascular, fractures of the shaft may result in excessive hemorrhage with loss of 1 or more liters of blood into the soft tissues of the thigh. Shock is usually present in varying degrees as a result of the injury and the associated blood loss.

The EMERGENCY TREATMENT of fracture of the femur is most important in securing a satisfactory end-result. No fracture except that of the cervical portion of the spine requires more care in the initial handling and transportation of the patient. If conscious, he will experience severe pain from any movement of the injured limb. The patient should be splinted where he falls at the time of the injury. For safe transportation a Thomas splint may be applied over the trousers, with traction by means of a twisted rope extending from a bandage or strap sling around the ankle. Unless there is evidence of an injury to the brain, morphine should be given before the patient is moved. If a Thomas splint is not available, a bed slat or other board which will reach from near the axilla to below the foot may be bandaged securely in place, after the leg is carefully straightened and aligned as gently as possible. A third method (and one which is

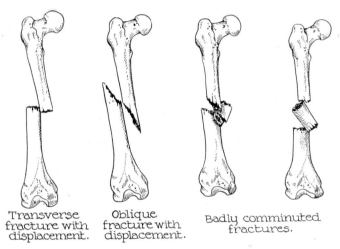

Transverse fracture with displacement.   Oblique fracture with displacement.   Badly comminuted fractures.

Fig. 155.—Types of fractures of the shaft of the femur.

moderately satisfactory) consists of bandaging the two lower extremities snugly together.

No patient who has sustained a serious injury to the femur should ever be picked up hastily, with thigh, knee and spine flexed, and placed in the rumble or back seat of an automobile. This is an ambulance case, and the patient should be kept at the place of injury until a stretcher can be provided or an ambulance obtained.

Fractures of the Shaft.—Fractures of the shaft of the femur in infants are treated by direct overhead traction applied

to both legs (Fig. 44). The infant should be actually lifted by
the suspension until no weight is borne on the back of the
sacrum. This same method is efficient in the treatment of children up to 7 or 8 years of age. For the older child and for the
adult, Russell traction is useful. The foot of the bed is elevated

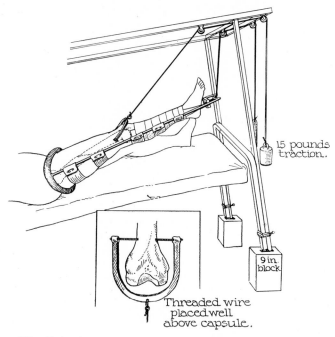

15 pounds
traction.

9 in.
block

Threaded wire
placed well
above capsule.

Fig. 156.—Skeletal traction for reduction of fractures of the shaft of the
femur.

and traction is applied only to the injured limb. The Boehler-
Braun splint or a Thomas splint, with or without Pierson attachment for flexion of the knee, adjusted skilfully until the lower
fragments line up with the upper fragments, will obtain a good
result provided sufficient traction is secured to reduce over-riding
and thus prevent shortening (Fig. 156). A threaded steel pin,

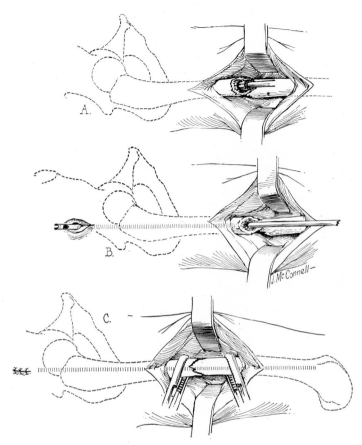

Fig. 157.—Introduction of an intramedullary rod into the femur by retrograde method. The fracture is exposed through lateral incision with the patient on the fracture table (Fig. 158). A stainless steel rod of correct size and length is driven upward through the medullary canal of the proximal fragment, so that the rod pierces the cortex of the neck just medial to the greater trochanter. A skin incision is made over the end of the rod where it presents in the gluteal region so it can emerge far enough for the other end of the rod to be introduced into the distal fragment. After the fracture is reduced, the rod is driven into the distal fragment to a level corresponding to the patella. A reamer, *A,* is used to enlarge the canal if it is too small to accept the rod or if it is obstructed by bone.

Steinmann pin or Kirschner wire inserted through the femur, high enough not to endanger the growth cartilage in children or the knee joint in either children or adults, provides a means for obtaining skeletal traction which is much more efficient than Buck's extension for fractures of this type.

For fractures of the midshaft junction of upper and middle

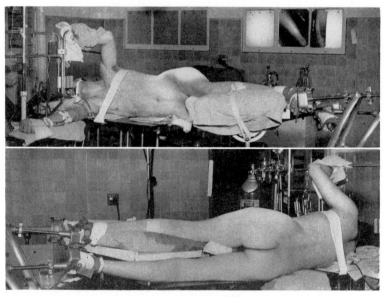

Fig. 158.—Positioning of the patient for introduction of an intramedullary rod into the femur. The feet are attached to the foot plates for support without traction.

thirds of the femur, the intramedullary rod is highly efficient (Figs. 157–159). It is the method of choice for the treatment of uncomplicated fractures of the shaft of the femur, except in those instances where comminution is so extensive that stability with the rod cannot be maintained.

When skilfully used, the method gives excellent immobilization, maintains the reduction and permits ambulation of the

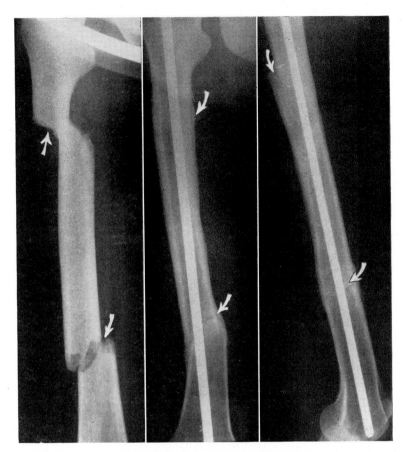

FIG. 159.—Segmental unstable fracture of the femur treated with an intramedullary rod, a method of internal fixation particularly suitable for such fractures.

301

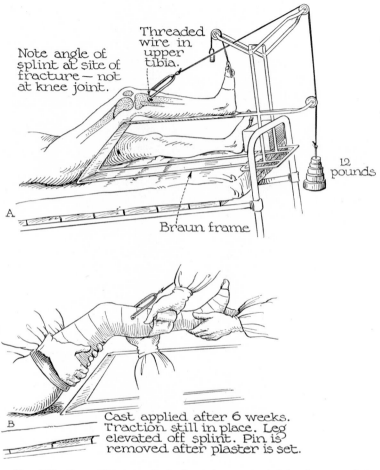

Note angle of splint at site of fracture — not at knee joint.

Threaded wire in upper tibia.

12 pounds

Braun frame

A

Cast applied after 6 weeks. Traction still in place. Leg elevated off splint. Pin is removed after plaster is set.

B

Fig. 160.—Braun frame method of treating supracondylar fracture of the femur.

302

patient, with active exercise of both the hip and the knee joint. From the standpoint of functional recovery and of obtaining reduction with a minimal cost for hospital care, this is the preferable method. Risk to the patient is undoubtedly greater than when only Buck's extension and Russell traction (or the Boehler-Braun or Thomas splint) are used. The method should be reserved for use by men who have had special training in fracture technique and who are sufficiently skilled to apply it without undue risk to the patient. Complications from the use of intra-

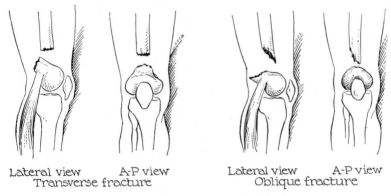

Lateral view   A-P view
Transverse fracture

Lateral view   A-P view
Oblique fracture

Fig. 161.—Posterior angulation of the condylar fragment of the femur produced by the pull of the gastrocnemius muscle.

medullary rods consist of upward or downward migration of the rod, bending or breaking of the rod, infection and splitting of the bone from too large a rod. These can be minimized by meticulous technique and proper execution of the procedure.

SUPRACONDYLAR FRACTURE of the femur which does not enter the knee joint may be successfully treated by traction, with a traction pin placed through the tibia just below the tuberosity and the knee maintained in a position of flexion on the Boehler-Braun splint, or a Thomas splint with Pierson attachment (Fig. 160). The backward angulation of the distal fragment, caused

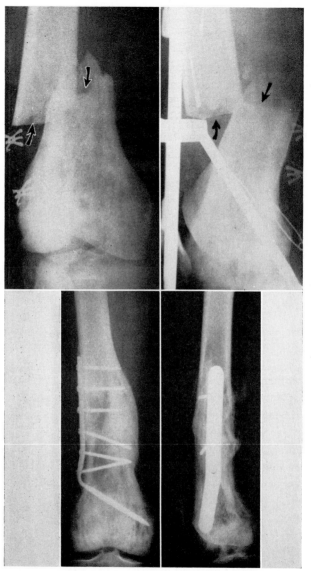

Fig. 162.—Fracture in the distal third of the femur through a region of typical osteitis deformans (Paget's disease) which was treated by an open reduction and immobilized by a blade plate. Closed reduction with skeletal traction was unsuccessful.

304

by spasm of the gastrocnemius muscle, is sometimes difficult to correct (Fig. 161). When the reduction has been obtained, traction must be maintained for at least four, and preferably six, weeks, when early callus can be demonstrated in the roentgenogram. A cast which is confined to the thigh and the lower leg may then be applied and the pin in the tibia may be incorporated to help maintain the reduction.

If treatment has been delayed, simple reduction may be difficult (Fig. 162). Direct upward traction on the distal femoral fragment by means of an additional Kirschner or threaded wire through the distal fragment at 90 degrees to the longitudinal axis of the femur may be necessary. Open reduction may be required, particularly if there is a T-fracture with displacement of the condyles.

DISPLACEMENT OF THE LOWER FEMORAL EPIPHYSIS occurs during childhood. It is in reality a slipping at the line of the epiphyseal growth cartilage plate. Most often the epiphysis is pushed anteriorly onto the anterior surface of the distal end of the shaft of the femur. Compression of the femoral artery and vein over the sharp edge of the distal end of the femoral diaphysis may result in serious circulatory disturbance of the foot. If the slip is not complete, reduction may be obtained by applying adhesive skin traction and extension of the leg. Dislocations of this type can also be reduced by manipulation under anesthesia. The procedure requires traction, with the knee held in flexion, and the reduction is maintained by immobilization of the leg with the knee flexed at approximately 90 degrees. When the swelling has subsided, after two to three weeks, the flexion can be gradually decreased. The cast should be changed every two weeks until complete extension is obtained. Since this injury occurs in children, there is little danger of permanent stiffness in the knee joint.

UNUNITED FRACTURE OF THE SHAFT of the femur may result from interposition of muscle between the fragments, extensive comminution, distraction of fragments or inadequate immobilization. When it occurs, an open operation is required. Any tissue which lies between the fracture ends should be removed

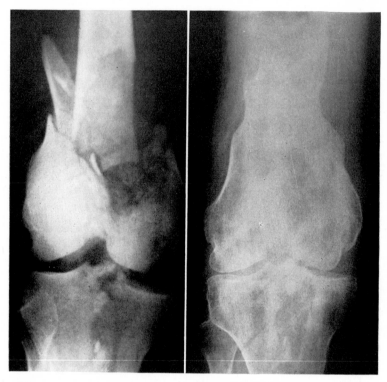

Fig. 163.—Severely comminuted fracture of distal end of femur and proximal tibia treated by skeletal traction with a pin through the distal third of the tibia. Excellent recovery of knee joint function was obtained.

and the bone ends freshened and approximated. Accurate apposition of the fragments with restoration of normal length should be obtained by means of direct traction on the fracture table or by manipulation. A full thickness tibial bone graft should then be onlaid. This graft should be of adequate length and as wide as can be obtained from the tibia of the patient without weakening this bone to the extent that fracture may occur. A metal plate with at least three screws above and three below the fracture will offer excellent assurance of maintaining alignment and preventing torsion. This may be applied directly over the antero-lateral surface of the femur while the onlay tibial bone graft is placed just posterior to the plate. Additional fragments of cancellous bone or osteoperiosteal bone should be packed around the line of fracture. A plaster cast, which includes the body, the entire leg and the opposite thigh, is then applied. Immobilization must be maintained until advanced union has occurred between the fracture fragments and between the graft and the femoral shaft. This period varies from four to six months.

We prefer to utilize an intramedullary rod for immobilization and thereby avoid the disadvantages of the hip spica cast whenever the location and nature of the nonunion will permit its insertion (Fig. 22). The bone ends are exposed and prepared, the rod is inserted by the retrograde method; the bone grafts are onlaid and secured in position by circumferential loops of chromic catgut, stainless steel wire or screws.

If, however, the alignment of the bone fragments is normal but union has failed to develop, the rod may be inserted by the direct method in which it is passed into the bone just medial to the tip of the greater trochanter and hammered down the intramedullary canal for the desired distance. Bone grafts are applied as previously described.

The MALUNITED FRACTURE OF THE SHAFT of the femur may include angulation with over-riding, producing deformity, shortening and permanent disability. Treatment for malunion consists of open reduction and application of bone grafts. A tourniquet may be applied at the groin to avoid bleeding and the attendant shock. To prevent it from slipping down into the field of operation, the tourniquet may be held in place by first inserting a Steinmann pin through the skin and fascia, in an anteroposterior direction, at the level of the tip of the greater trochanter. If the tourniquet is applied around the thigh and carried up over the ends of this pin, it will accomplish its purpose with safety and efficiency. Blood transfusions must be given during the operation as an additional measure of safety.

The old fracture line should be opened up by means of sharp osteotomes. If the over-riding is marked, it may be difficult to restore the full length. Shortened muscles do not respond to immediate traction stretch, and care should be taken not to tear major blood vessels. In most instances, however, a gradual stretch on the fracture table will bring about restoration of length when the shortening has not exceeded $1\frac{1}{2}$ in.

The femoral fragments should be carefully realigned, the rotation corrected and an intramedullary rod or metal plate used to secure the position. An onlay tibial bone graft, such as that used for any case of nonunion, with additional fragments of cancellous or osteoperiosteal bone from the tibia or ilium packed around the fracture line, will markedly improve the chances of solid union in the usual period of time. This is a formidable procedure and should not be attempted by an inexperienced surgeon.

CHAPTER XXVI

The Knee

INJURIES of the knee include fractures of the patella, the condyles of the femur and the tibial spines and plateaus. Dislocation of the knee is exceedingly rare. When it occurs it must be preceded by rupture of the cruciate ligaments and usually includes tear and displacement of the semilunar cartilages.

FRACTURES OF THE PATELLA.—These may be closed, open, transverse or comminuted. The patella is covered on its joint surface by articular hyaline cartilage. Unless the alignment of this bone is accurately restored, an irregular surface will persist following healing of the fracture. This produces arthritis of the knee joint by friction and erosion, as the roughened patella traverses the femoral groove in flexion and extension of the knee. Arthritic disability following this fracture is so common that certain authors recommend total excision of the patella in all fractures with separation of fragments. Transverse fractures with the proximal and distal fragments of approximately equal size should be accurately reduced and immobilized until union occurs. Comminuted fragments should be excised, and if a major portion or all is involved total excision is advisable (Fig. 164).

An *incomplete fracture of the patella,* consisting only of a crack without separation of fragments, is treated by a skin-tight plaster cast cylinder from the groin to just above the ankle,

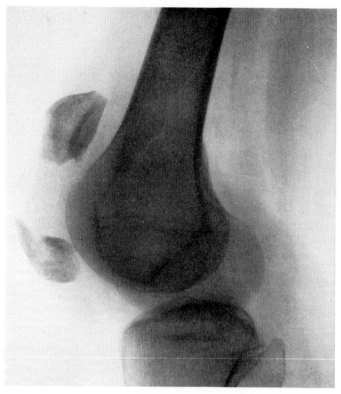

Fig. 164.—For fractures of the patella with asymmetrical fragments and separation we recommend excision of lesser fragments and suture of the quadriceps tendon or infrapatellar ligament with chromic catgut or fine wire to the major fragment. Relaxed motion may be permitted after three weeks and unrestricted activity after two months.

molded firmly over the condyles of the femur to prevent slipping downward (Fig. 165). The patient should be encouraged to walk with crutches and after three weeks to begin full weight-bearing. The cast should be worn for no less than six weeks.

A *transverse fracture* with wide separation of fragments is always associated with tearing of the knee joint capsule on both sides. In such injuries the joint space is filled with blood. This type of injury can be treated satisfactorily only by open operation. It is not an emergency and the operation may be delayed until the acute local traumatic reaction has subsided and all

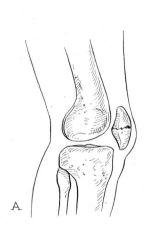

A

Transverse fracture
of patella without
separation of fragments.

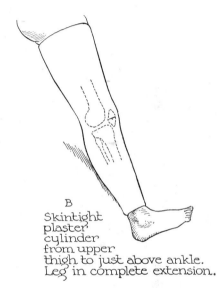

B
Skintight
plaster
cylinder
from upper
thigh to just above ankle.
Leg in complete extension.

Fig. 165.

abrasions have healed. During this interval the leg should be supported in a posterior splint and kept elevated. A transverse incision affords the best exposure (Fig. 166). The blood clot and all small fragments of bone found in the joint should be removed and the joint surfaces sponged clean with warm, soft, moist sponges. The capsule should be repaired with no. 2 chromic catgut sutures. The fracture surfaces of the patella are accurately approximated and held in position by a heavy braided silk or

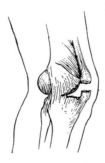

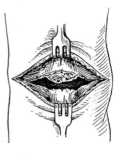

A

Transverse fracture
of patella with tear
of capsule and sep-
aration of fragments

B

Transverse incision
exposing fracture
and torn capsule

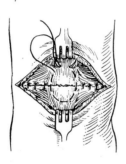

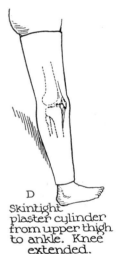

C

Capsule sutured.
Fracture reduced
and maintained by
circumferential
loop of heavy silk

D

Skintight
plaster cylinder
from upper thigh
to ankle. Knee
extended.

FIG. 166.—Purse-string suture for fracture of the patella.

steel wire suture passed completely around the two fragments to hold them together. A plaster cast cylinder from the groin to above the ankle should then be applied and worn for six weeks. The patient may be ambulatory, with crutches, but no weight should be borne on the foot of the injured limb for three weeks. Physical therapy and active motion should be started six weeks after injury. The cast may be bivalved and re-applied after each

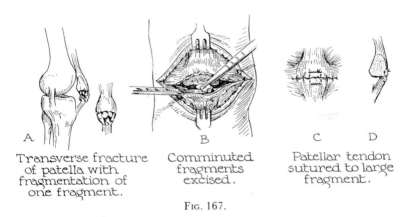

Transverse fracture of patella with fragmentation of one fragment.

Comminuted fragments excised.

Patellar tendon sutured to large fragment.

A   B   C   D

FIG. 167.

treatment for an additional period of two weeks or until muscular control of the knee has been regained.

Comminuted fractures with one large fragment and several small fragments are treated by excision of the small fragments. The quadriceps tendon or the infrapatellar ligament should be sutured to the large fragment with heavy silk or wire passed through drill holes in the bone (Fig. 167). If the patella is extensively comminuted and there is no major intact fragment, all fragments should be excised and the infrapatellar ligament sutured securely to the quadriceps tendon (Fig. 168). The advantage of using wire rather than any other suture material lies in the fact that quadriceps setting exercises may be started early with less danger of separation. Avulsion of either the quadriceps

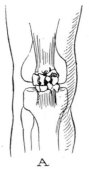

A

Badly comminuted
fracture of patella.

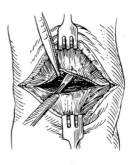

B

Patellar fragments
excised subperiosteally

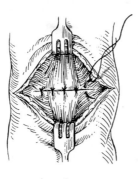

C

Quadriceps tendon.
and patellar tendon.
sutured together.
Torn capsule repaired.

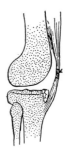

D

Cross-section
showing
sutured
tendons.

Fig. 168.

tendon or the patellar ligament with a small bone fragment
should be treated by removal of the small fragment and suturing with wire (Figs. 169 and 170).

FRACTURES OF THE CONDYLES OF THE FEMUR.—These may
be reduced by manipulation and traction assisted by molding
the fragments with the hands. Harsh compression with a bone

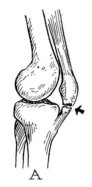

A

Avulsion of
patellar
tendon

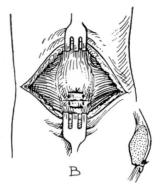

B

Excise fragment
and suture patellar
tendon to front
of patella

Fig. 169.

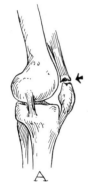

A

Avulsion of
quadriceps
tendon.

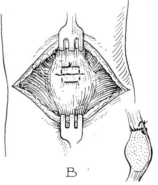

B

Excise small upper
bone fragment and
suture tendon to
front of patella.

Fig. 170.

clamp should not be necessary and may produce severe contusion and bruising. Markedly comminuted fractures of the distal end of the femur, including the articular surfaces, can be molded into surprisingly good position by continuous traction, using a threaded steel wire or pin through the tibia just below the tuberosity. The knee is held in 45 degree flexion on a Boehler-Braun frame or a Thomas splint with Pierson attachment. The advantage of the Pierson attachment lies in the fact that it permits early knee joint motion. If adequate reduction is not obtained by traction or closed manipulation, open reduction with fixation of the fragments with a metal flange, metal screws or threaded wires is necessary. One or both cruciate ligaments may be ruptured and even when surgical repair cannot be accomplished, the result may be satisfactory if the reduction is adequate and the quadriceps power is restored by proper resistive exercises.

FRACTURES OF THE TIBIA which extend into the knee joint include those of the tibial spines and of the tuberosities of the tibia. The anterior cruciate ligament is attached to the anterior tibial spine and may be avulsed at the time of injury with detachment of the spine. Occasionally the fragment may be satisfactorily reduced by complete extension of the knee. If the fragment cannot be replaced and maintained in position by a circular plaster dressing, an open operation should be performed. *The fragment should not be removed.* It is accurately replaced, a no. 2 chromic suture is passed through the cruciate ligament at the tip of the spinous process and brought forward through two drill holes in the adjacent tibia and tied between the drill holes. The leg should be immobilized in a snug plaster cylinder for six weeks (Fig. 171).

FRACTURES OF THE TIBIAL PLATEAUS.—The weight of the body is transmitted from the femur onto the proximal broadened articular surfaces of the tibia. Fractures of either tibial plateau or of the femoral condyles may be produced by direct violence in which the femoral condyles are driven into the contiguous articulating surfaces of the tibia. Both tibial plateaus may be fractured simultaneously in a fall from a height. More often the lateral condyle is broken by direct trauma to the lateral aspect of the knee, such as occurs when a pedestrian is struck by the bumper of an automobile. The resulting fracture may be one of two types. The fracture may begin near the tibial spine and extend downward and outward with depression of the entire lateral condyle (Fig. 172). In other instances there is a greater

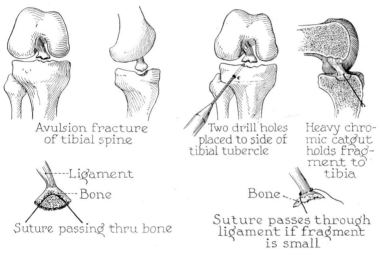

Avulsion fracture of tibial spine

Ligament
Bone
Suture passing thru bone

Two drill holes placed to side of tibial tubercle

Heavy chromic catgut holds fragment to tibia

Bone

Suture passes through ligament if fragment is small

Fig. 171.—Treatment of avulsion fracture of tibial spine.

degree of valgus of the knee and the force is transmitted through the sharp outer margin of the lateral femoral condyle to the central weight-bearing surface of the corresponding half of the tibial plateau (Figs. 173 and 174). This may produce a comminuted fracture of the joint surface. The tibial articular fragments will be impacted and driven downward into the cancellous bone of the upper end of the tibia. The lateral cortex may also be displaced outward, and frequently the lateral semilunar cartilage is torn and embedded in the comminuted bone. The

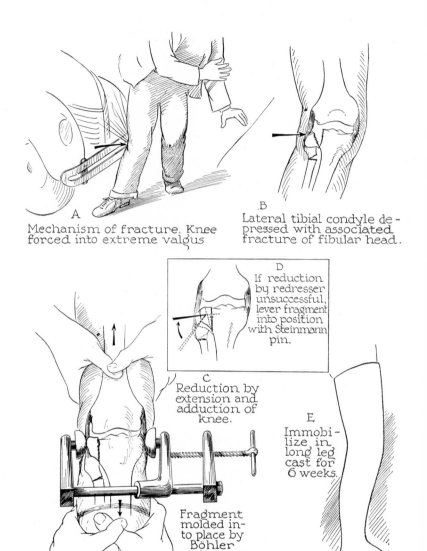

A
Mechanism of fracture. Knee
forced into extreme valgus

B
Lateral tibial condyle depressed with associated
fracture of fibular head.

D
If reduction
by redresser
unsuccessful,
lever fragment
into position
with Steinmann
pin.

C
Reduction by
extension and
adduction of
knee.

E
Immobi-
lize in
long leg
cast for
6 weeks.

Fragment
molded in-
to place by
Böhler
redresser.

Fig. 172.—The bumper fracture of the condyle of the tibia.

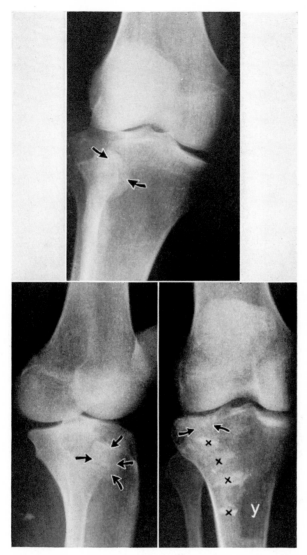

Fig. 173.—Depressed fracture of the lateral plateau of the tibia without separation of a large fragment. The depressed fragments (arrows) should be elevated through a window, *y*, resulting from removal of a tibial bone graft. Bone, ×, from the tibia is then wedged beneath the elevated plateau to maintain it in the reduced position.

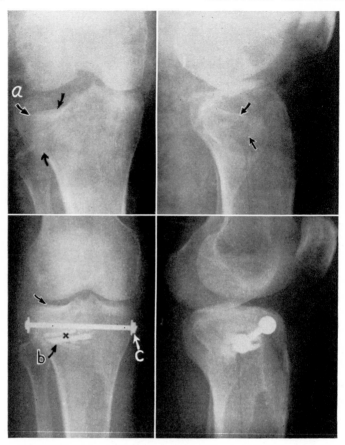

Fig. 174.—Depressed fracture of the lateral plateau of the tibia, *a*. The depressed fragments were elevated and supported with bone grafts taken from the medial cortex of the tibia, *b*, and the major fragments maintained in position with a tibial bolt, *c*.

medial collateral ligament may be partially or completely torn. This added injury may be overlooked because of the valgus deformity of the knee which is primarily due to the depression of the articular surface.

The medial plateau is less frequently fractured, because the inner aspect of the knee is less exposed to direct violence. The principles of treatment are the same as for fractures of the lateral plateau.

Fractures of both tibial plateaus without displacement may be treated by a long leg plaster cast for six weeks with the patient ambulatory on crutches. The shoe of the well leg should be elevated $\frac{1}{2}$ in. Fractures with slight displacement should be reduced as shown in Figure 174. The leg should be placed in direct traction on the fracture table with the patient under a general anesthetic. The condyles may be molded into position, either manually or with a well padded bone clamp. A plaster cylinder should be applied after a Kirschner or threaded wire has been passed through the distal third of the tibia. Skeletal traction should be maintained for six weeks. A single hip spica cast may be applied for an additional six weeks and the patient permitted to be ambulatory on crutches. Prolonged physical therapy and full co-operation of the patient will be required to mobilize the knee and restore quadriceps power. If the joint surface of the tibia cannot be accurately restored by closed treatment, the patient is entitled to an open reduction. The fragments are replaced accurately and fixed by means of multiple threaded wires or a Barr bolt. Active motion is resumed after three weeks, but weight-bearing must not be attempted for three months.

Fractures with displacement of the entire lateral plateau are reduced by traction and the use of a redresser. A long leg cast should be worn for six weeks. This should be followed by physical therapy. Weight-bearing may be resumed gradually after 12 weeks. Open reduction becomes necessary when adequate reposition of the fragment cannot be accomplished by closed methods. The fragment is elevated into position and fixed with threaded wires or a bolt. Motion should be resumed after three weeks, but otherwise the postoperative course is the same as following closed reduction.

A third type of fracture, in which there is definite depression of the central surface of the lateral plateau, requires surgical reconstruction (Figs. 173 and 174). Closed reduction cannot elevate the impacted, depressed bone or reduce the torn and

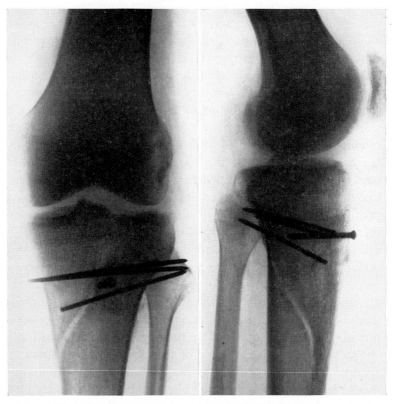

FIG. 175.—Spiral fracture of proximal end of the tibia. Open reduction. Lateral semilunar cartilage found displaced deep between the fracture fragments was removed. Accurate reduction and fixation with threaded pins resulted in healing with good anatomic and excellent functional results.

displaced lateral semilunar cartilage. This reconstruction is difficult and the results are often not satisfactory even when performed by the experienced orthopedic surgeon. However, unless the plateau is restored and the level of the weight-bearing sur-

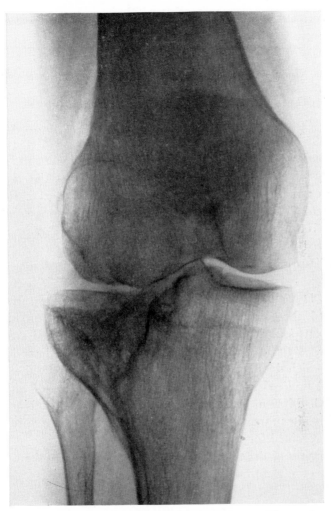

Fig. 176.—Malunion of fracture of the tibial plateau. The persistent depression of the lateral weight-bearing surface of approximately ½ in. caused pain and instability. These fractures are best treated by open reduction, accurate alignment of joint surfaces, fixation by threaded pins or bolt and removal of displaced semilunar cartilages and repair of torn ligaments.

face corrected, the knee will be unstable from side to side and permanent use of a long leg brace may be necessary.

The knee joint, lateral condyle and the proximal fourth of the medial subcutaneous surface of the tibia must be exposed for an open reduction.

A lateral parapatellar incision is extended downward over the anterior surface of the lateral condyle of the tibia and is curved medially below the tubercle to end over the crest of the tibia. The knee joint is opened and the lateral semilunar cartilage is usually removed, regardless of its appearance. This gives a complete exposure of the articular surfaces. A bone graft 2½ in. long and ¾ in. wide is removed distal to the tibial tubercle, and access is thus gained to the interior of the tibia. A large impactor is passed upward through the opening so that it contacts the cancellous bone beneath the depressed fracture fragments. The articular surface is elevated by means of a mallet striking the end of the impactor projecting from the tibia. After the surface is restored, the bone graft which was removed is split into several fragments and these are impacted beneath the restored articular bone. A Barr bolt may be used if there is a large lateral fragment which does not otherwise hold in satisfactory position. The wound is closed in layers and a loosely padded long leg cast is applied. Motion is permitted after four weeks and weightbearing after three months. Maximum motion in the knee joint is not regained for four to six months.

Fractures of the tibial plateau with malunion may be treated by osteotomy and reconstruction of the joint surface or by arthrodesis if the disruption is too great to justify an attempt to salvage a mobile joint.

Fracture of the tibial tubercle or epiphyseal separation which occurs in adolescents may be treated conservatively by a plaster of paris dressing from groin to ankle. Marked *separation of the tubercle,* as in some avulsion fractures, needs open operation, accurate replacement and fixation with metal screws or sutures.

CHAPTER XXVII

The Leg

OF the two bones of the leg, the fibula rarely offers any real problem from the standpoint of fracture therapy. The fibula splints the larger weight-bearing bone and helps to re-enforce and stabilize the foot at the ankle. Isolated fractures in the proximal three fourths of the fibula do not require immobilization for healing. The patient may, however, be more comfortable in a short leg plaster cylinder or cast including the foot for 10–14 days, after which full function is quickly recovered. Fractures of the distal fourth of the fibula are usually associated with injuries at the ankle and they must be treated adequately. This usually means a cast for six to 10 weeks. These fractures are discussed in detail in Chapter XXVIII.

Of all the major bones in the human skeleton, the tibia is the least protected by soft tissue. Its entire antero-medial surface is covered by skin, subcutaneous fascia and periosteum. It is subject to injury from direct violence and also from torsion strains. Because it is so superficial in its anterior and medial aspects, fractures of the tibia are frequently open, and they are more often spiral or oblique than transverse.

STABLE FRACTURES OF THE SHAFT OF THE TIBIA.—For the purpose of treatment, fractures of the tibia may be classified as

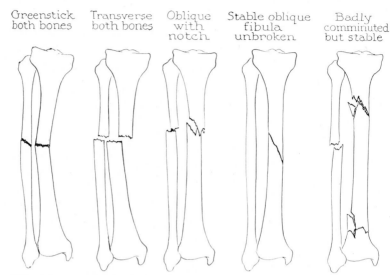

Greenstick both bones   Transverse both bones   Oblique with notch   Stable oblique fibula unbroken   Badly comminuted but stable

STABLE FRACTURES of TIBIA TREATED by PLASTER CAST

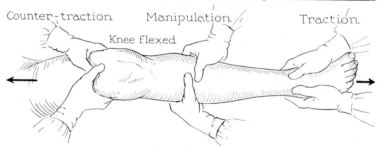

Counter-traction   Manipulation   Traction

Knee flexed

Follow reduction with cast from ankle to upper thigh. After cast sets, include foot. Pad bony prominences, and allow space for swelling.

FIG. 177.—Fractures of the tibia which may be treated successfully by plaster cast.

stable or unstable. The first can ordinarily be treated conservatively by closed reduction and a plaster cast, while the latter require continuous traction or a surgical re-position.

Stable fractures of the tibia may be transverse, with or without displacement; short oblique fractures but notched so that they remain aligned once the fragments are engaged, and undisplaced oblique fractures with the fibula intact so that leg length is maintained.

Stable fractures of the tibia should be accurately reduced to restore length and to correct any torsion which may disturb the normal relationship between the knee and the ankle joint (Fig. 177). If there is no displacement of the fracture fragments, a plaster cast from the groin to and including the foot will help to protect against over-riding or loss of apposition of the fragments. If the fracture is transverse, with over-riding or with torsion, reduction should be attempted by manual traction, with the knee flexed 90 degrees over the end of a fracture table or on a fracture table.

UNSTABLE FRACTURES OF THE SHAFTS OF THE TIBIA AND FIBULA.—If the fracture is definitely oblique and there are no fragments which can be interlocked, it is not possible to maintain length and adequate bone contact by plaster cast alone.

Three avenues of treatment are available to the physician. These are skeletal traction, multiple pin fixation and open reduction. Circumstances presented by different patients may dictate the utilization of one method rather than another. A pin for skeletal traction may be placed through the distal portion of the tibia or the os calcis, depending on the location of the fracture, with the leg suspended on a Thomas splint. Over-riding is easily corrected but it is difficult to get side-to-side compression at the site of fracture. Traction is continued, if the reduction is satisfactory, until there is early roentgen evidence of callus. This does not occur before six weeks. A long leg cast is then applied and the patient may be ambulatory on crutches.

Multiple pin fixation is less popular than it was several years ago, but in properly selected cases one may have quite satisfactory results. One threaded wire or pin may be passed through the tibia about 1 in. above the ankle joint, a drill being used for this purpose (Fig. 178). A second pin should be drilled through the tibia just below the level of the tibial tuberosity. Reduction

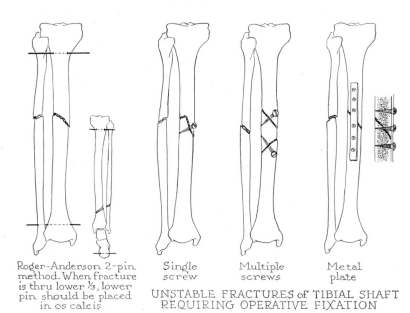

Roger-Anderson 2-pin method. When fracture is thru lower ⅓, lower pin should be placed in os calcis.

Single screw

Multiple screws

Metal plate

UNSTABLE FRACTURES of TIBIAL SHAFT REQUIRING OPERATIVE FIXATION

Fig. 178.

is obtained by traction on the fracture table or the leg is held in a vertical position over the end of the table, with the knee flexed 90 degrees. A plaster cast with minimal padding should be applied from the groin to the toes. Both pins are incorporated in the cast. While the plaster is setting, the surgeon should carefully adjust the fragments to obtain maximal position. The patient is returned to bed and the leg is elevated on pillows. The patient is permitted to walk with the aid of crutches as soon as the circulation is satisfactory.

If alignment of the tibia is not satisfactory in subsequent roentgenograms, this may be improved by *wedging the cast* (Fig. 179). The wedge is executed by cutting the plaster cast

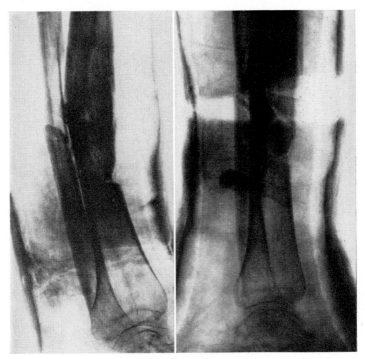

Fig. 179.—Plaster cast wedging.

two thirds of the way around, several inches above the site of angulation. When the cast is then opened, a corrective force will be directed toward the deformity.

Open reduction and internal fixation by means of multiple screws or a metal plate, depending on the obliquity of the bone ends, is the third method of treating unstable tibial fractures.

Infections are infrequent but, when they do occur, are serious complications of surgical reductions. There is little doubt that union is delayed by the surgical trauma, and nonunion may result from this surgical insult. For these reasons the surgeon

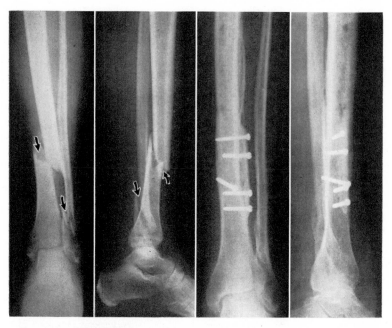

FIG. 180.—Oblique fracture of the tibia through the junction of the middle and distal thirds with an oblique comminuted fracture of the distal third of the fibula. The oblique fracture was transfixed with one screw. A full-thickness bone graft from the adjacent tibia was transfixed with four stainless steel screws. This method is indicated particularly when there has been a delay of three or four weeks in reduction of the fracture.

must be meticulous in his technique to avoid an infection, and the use of a primary onlay bone graft obtained from the same tibia to stimulate osteogenesis is excellent surgical treatment. A long leg cast is routinely applied for external fixation. An alternative method of casting which does not immobilize the knee can be used. Two threaded wires are placed through the proximal third of the tibia near the tuberosity and these wires are incorporated in a below-the-knee cast, with nuts and washers on the wire ends to maintain tautness. Figure 180 illustrates a fracture treated in this manner.

Immobilization should be continued until the roentgenograms show positive evidence of union, irrespective of the method of

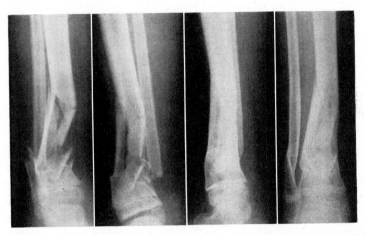

Fig. 181.—Extensively comminuted fracture of the distal third of the tibia and fibula. A fracture with such severe comminution, particularly in a growing child, is best treated conservatively. In this instance, traction through the heel was maintained for six weeks, followed by immobilization in a long leg plaster cast for two months. Open surgery would have contributed to vascular deficiency in the multiple bone fragments.

reduction. Weight-bearing without protection of the cast is permitted only after union has occurred. The total period of disability following fractures of the middle third of the tibia, with or without associated fractures of the fibula, and when there are no postreduction complications, is rarely less than five months, and one year may be required for complete functional recovery. Fractures at the level of the lower and middle thirds may disrupt the blood supply and cause a marked delay in union. Most of these fractures will heal, however, if the plaster cast maintains immobilization and is continued for a long enough time (Fig. 181). A full year may be required before there is sufficient roentgenographic and clinical evidence of healing to permit unprotected weight-bearing if major nutrient blood vessels have been ruptured.

Segmental fractures are treated best by open reduction and internal fixation, when there is instability at one or both fracture sites.

OPEN FRACTURES of the tibia or fibula should be treated as described in Chapter XI. If the patient is seen within eight hours after the injury, the wound should be cleansed thoroughly with soap and water, débrided and then washed out with normal saline. The surgeon may then use a long leg cast or, if the fracture is oblique, the fragments may be held securely by two stainless steel screws passed completely through the cortex of each fragment. Another satisfactory method of maintaining position of the fragments makes use of a metal plate, using three screws in each fragment (Fig. 13). With the wound already opened, accurate reduction can be obtained readily under visual control. The wound should be closed without suturing fascia, using silk for the skin but permitting enough distance between each suture to allow for drainage.

In NONUNION of fractures of both bones of the leg, the fibula can be ignored. (This applies to acute closed fractures also.) For nonunion of the tibia, a bone graft may be cut from the major fragment and used as an inlay or onlay graft across the fracture line. Such grafts should be large and should be re-enforced with additional osteoperiosteal or cancellous bone placed around the line of fracture.

The treatment of INFECTED FRACTURES of the tibia is the same as that of infected fractures or chronic osteomyelitis elsewhere. Devitalized fragments of bone or definite sequestra are removed. All infected tissue that can be definitely identified is also cleaned from the wound. The position of the fragments is improved as much as possible without forced manipulation. The wound should be spread open with loose folds of petrolatum gauze. The cast should extend from the groin to the base of the toes and must not be windowed. Unless the drainage is excessive or the odor extreme, the cast should not be changed more often than once in six weeks. The appropriate antibiotic should be used after sensitivity tests have been run on cultures from the wound. A bone graft will be required to obtain union if healing fails to occur.

CHAPTER XXVIII

The Ankle

THE ankle joint is formed by the articulation of the astragalus with the distal ends of the tibia and fibula. In addition, there is a small but distinct joint between the tibia and the fibula, just proximal to the ankle joint, that frequently communicates directly with the primary joint space. Stability of the ankle is dependent upon the continuity of the ligaments and maintenance of the mortise formed by the tibia and fibula. The malleoli limit medial, lateral and rotary motion of the foot on the leg. Fractures which alter these relationships must be accurately reduced if the patient is to recover normal use of the ankle. Inadequate reduction with instability leads invariably to traumatic arthritis.

Injuries to the ankle consist of varying combinations of fractures of the distal articular surface of the tibia, the malleoli and the astragalus; dislocations of the astragalar-tibial-fibular joint, and sprains of either the internal or the lateral ligaments.

FRACTURES OF THE ANKLE have been divided into specific groups according to the direction into which the foot is displaced by the injury. *Abduction* fractures occur when the foot is directed outward (into *valgus*) by a force applied to the lateral aspect of the leg or the medial side of the foot. When the foot is forcibly directed medially (into *varus*), a so-called *adduction* fracture results. In a pure abduction or adduction fracture either both malleoli are broken *(bimalleolar fracture)* or one malleolus is fractured and the opposite collateral ligament is ruptured or partly torn. Ordinarily, additional forces come into play in these two main types of ankle fractures. If the injury which forces the foot into marked abduction or adduction also causes the foot to be directed backward, a fracture of the posterior lip of the articular surface of the tibia may occur with or without a posterior dislocation of the foot to a varying degree. A fracture involving both malleoli as well as the posterior surface of the tibia *(posterior malleolus)* is known as a *trimalleolar* or Cotton fracture. On the other hand, when the fracture force thrusts the foot forward on the tibia, the anterior lip of the tibia may be fractured, along with one or both malleoli.

Rotational force through the ankle joint mortise produces oblique rather than transverse fractures of the malleoli, although the combinations of fractures and ligamentous injuries are similar to those of the abduction or adduction injuries.

Force directed downward through the tibia onto the foot may result in a fracture of the os calcis. Not infrequently, when the calcaneus is spared, there occurs a severely comminuted fracture of the distal articular surface of the tibia.

The treatment of ankle fractures is simplified if the physician will analyze the component parts of any given fracture and the forces which created them. Reduction is accomplished by manipulations which reverse these forces.

ABDUCTION FRACTURES OF THE ANKLE.—As the foot is forced into abduction, the lateral surface of the body of the astragalus compresses the medial aspect of the lateral malleolus and the internal (deltoid) ligament is placed under tension. If the deforming force stops here, there may occur a sprain of the deltoid ligament. More frequently the astragalus continues its outward path and knocks off the lateral malleolus by direct contact. The

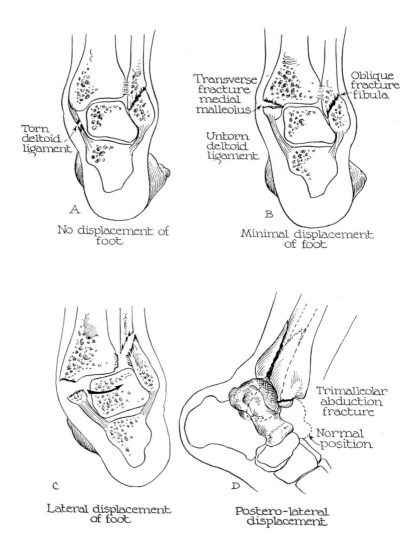

Fig. 182.—Eversion or abduction fractures of the ankle.

336

fracture of the fibula will be oblique if the foot also rotates in a clockwise direction. The deltoid ligament may rupture but is more likely to remain intact and produce an avulsion fracture of the medial malleolus. Posterior or posterior-lateral dislocation of the foot, with or without a fracture of the posterior malleolus, may occur as the force expends itself. Abduction injuries of the ankle may produce the following combinations of fractures (Fig. 182):

1. Fracture of the lateral malleolus.
2. Fracture of the lateral malleolus and rupture of the deltoid ligament.
3. Fracture of the medial and lateral malleoli *(bimalleolar or Pott's fracture)*.
4. Fracture of medial, lateral and posterior malleoli *(trimalleolar or Cotton fracture)*.
5. Any combination of the foregoing with lateral or posterior-lateral dislocation of the foot.

The diagnosis of an abduction fracture is seldom difficult to make. The history of an abduction injury followed by pain, loss of function of the ankle, swelling, tenderness over the malleoli, with or without lateral displacement of the foot, will indicate a fracture of the ankle joint. Roentgenograms taken in the antero-posterior, lateral and oblique views will disclose the exact nature of the fracture.

TREATMENT OF ABDUCTION FRACTURES

Simple fractures of the lateral malleolus without displacement should be immobilized for four weeks in a short leg cast in which a walking iron may be incorporated for early weight-bearing. If the malleolus is displaced laterally to even a slight degree, accurate reduction must be obtained to restore the joint mortise to its normal position. Bimalleolar abduction or Pott's fractures may be reduced as illustrated in Figure 183. The anesthesia of choice is Pentothal sodium intravenously, although procaine may be injected into the fracture sites. Flex the knee to 90 degrees while an assistant applies countertraction by pulling up on the tibia. Grasp the foot by the heel and forefoot and apply downward traction, while molding the foot medially and forward under the tibia. The foot should be dorsiflexed to 90 degrees and forced into sufficient varus as a short leg cast is applied. The ankle joint mortise is restored to normal by molding the plaster

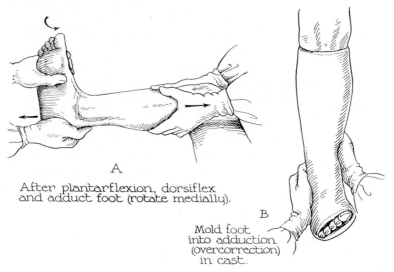

A.

After plantarflexion, dorsiflex
and adduct foot (rotate medially).

B

Mold foot
into adduction
(overcorrection)
in cast.

FIG. 183.—Treatment of eversion fracture of the ankle.

over the malleoli with the flat of the hands and compressing them together. A pad of felt over the malleoli and heel will help to prevent pain or necrosis from pressure. If the patient complains of pain over a bony prominence, the cast should be windowed to relieve the pressure. Until the cast dries keep the patient in bed with the foot elevated on a pillow to reduce the swelling. Check-up roentgenograms should be taken; and if the reduction is not accurate, it must be repeated as many times as is necessary to obtain exact re-position of the fragments. Persistent lateral displacement of the astragalus of no more than ¼ in. is very likely to lead to degenerative changes and permanent disability in this weight-bearing joint. Frequently the medial malleolus is widely displaced and cannot be restored to its normal position. Open reduction and internal fixation of the malleolar fragment is then indicated (Fig. 184). It is unnecessary to obtain anatomic reduction of the fibular fracture unless the intra-articular portion of the lateral malleolus happens to be involved.

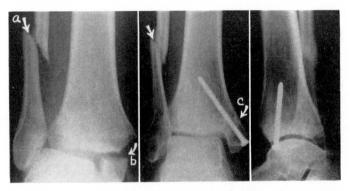

FIG. 184.—Fracture of distal third of fibula, *a,* and medial malleolus, *b,* with moderate displacement of the malleolar fragment. When closed reduction does not maintain accurate position of a large medial malleolar fragment, open reduction and accurate internal fixation of the medial malleolus with a stainless steel screw is definitely to be recommended, *c.* As a rule, the fibular fracture requires no special attention.

A snug-fitting cast is required to maintain the reduction. The original plaster dressing usually becomes loose after seven to 10 days as the swelling subsides and a new snug-fitting cast must be applied. Roentgenograms should be obtained to determine the position of the fragments after each cast change. After reduction of the fracture, the patient may be permitted to be ambulatory with the aid of crutches. We do not advise weight-bearing in the cast except in isolated undisplaced or otherwise stable fractures of the malleoli. Roentgenograms should be taken at six weeks; and if there is evidence of union, the cast may be removed. If there is insufficient callus around the fracture, the cast should be continued for another four weeks, at which time roentgenograms are repeated.

Normal function should be achieved within four to six months from the time of injury if reduction is accurate and union is solid. Physical therapy will hasten recovery of motion of the foot and ankle. Full weight-bearing may be permitted as tolerated by the patient.

Trimalleolar (Cotton) fractures may be reduced by the same technique described for bimalleolar fractures with dislocation of the foot. The foot must be immobilized in extreme dorsiflexion to tighten the posterior capsule of the ankle and hold down the posterior lip fragment of the tibia to which the capsule is attached. Maximal dorsiflexion of the foot is obtained with the knee flexed to 90 degrees to relax the Achilles tendon. Tibial fragments containing one fourth or more of the articular surface must be accurately replaced to restore the continuity of the joint surface and prevent recurrent posterior dislocation of the foot. Open reduction and fixation of the fragment by metal screws is indicated if accurate reposition cannot be accomplished by manipulation. Smaller fragments are unimportant unless they encroach on the joint. The postreduction treatment is the same as for Pott's fractures, but weight-bearing should be delayed for 10 weeks after reduction of the fracture.

ADDUCTION FRACTURES OF THE ANKLE JOINT.—Adduction fractures are produced by a force which drives the astragalus medially against the medial malleolus and places the lateral ligament of the ankle under tension (Fig. 185). If the force is checked here, only a sprain of the ankle may result. On the other hand, if the force continues, any one of the following combinations of fractures may result:

1. Simple fracture of the medial malleolus.
2. Fracture, with medial displacement, of the medial malleo-

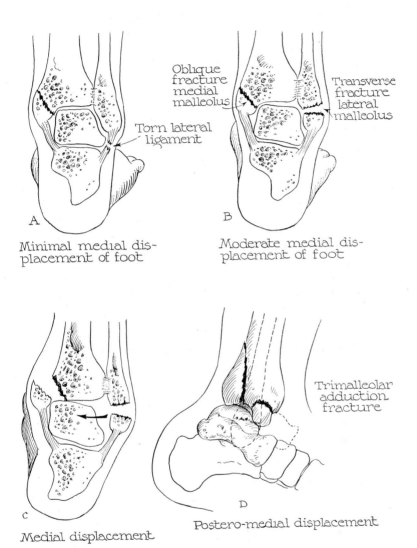

Oblique fracture medial malleolus

Transverse fracture lateral malleolus

Torn lateral ligament

A

Minimal medial displacement of foot

B

Moderate medial displacement of foot

Trimalleolar adduction fracture

C

Medial displacement

D

Postero-medial displacement

Fig. 185.—Inversion or adduction fractures of the ankle.

341

lus and rupture of the lateral ligament or avulsion of the lateral malleolus.

3. Fracture of the medial, lateral and posterior malleoli with dislocation of the foot (Cotton type).

Treatment of adduction fractures of the ankle is similar to that described for abduction fractures, but the directions of the forces applied in the manipulations are reversed. After downward traction on the foot, the dislocation may be corrected by bringing the foot beneath the tibia, and a short leg cast should be applied while molding the malleoli and maintaining at least 90 degree dorsiflexion of the foot (Fig. 186). Occasionally it will be necessary to plantar flex the foot before applying downward and forward traction in order to clear the astragalus from the posterior surface of the tibia when there is marked posterior and proximal dislocation. The postreduction treatment consists of cast immobilization for six to 10 weeks followed by physical therapy and gradual weight-bearing. The importance of accurate reduction of ankle joint fractures must again be emphasized. A poor reduction will not result in the restoration of normal ankle function.

FRACTURES OF ANTERIOR MARGIN OF DISTAL ARTICULAR SURFACE OF THE TIBIA.—When the foot is dislocated anteriorly instead of posteriorly as an isolated injury or in conjunction with an abduction or adduction fracture of the ankle, a fragment of varying size may be sheared from the distal anterior margin of the tibia. Accurate reposition may be obtained by manipulation. The anterior dislocation of the foot reduces without difficulty, and the tibial fragment should then be molded into position. Plantar flexion of the foot may be necessary to pull the fragment down through the medium of the attachments of the anterior capsule. The foot should be immobilized in the reduced position for six weeks. Open reduction will be required when there is no prospect that adequate reduction can be obtained by the closed method.

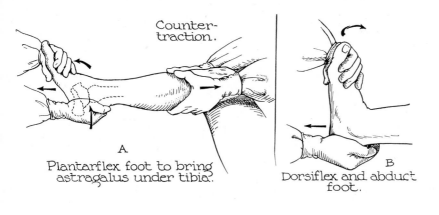

Counter-traction.

A

Plantarflex foot to bring astragalus under tibia.

B

Dorsiflex and abduct foot.

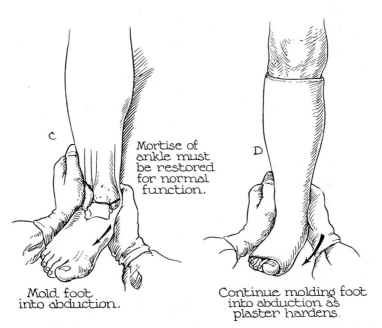

C

Mortise of ankle must be restored for normal function.

D

Mold foot into abduction.

Continue molding foot into abduction as plaster hardens.

FIG. 186.—Reduction and immobilization of inversion bimalleolar fracture.

COMMINUTED FRACTURES OF DISTAL ARTICULAR SURFACE OF
THE TIBIA.—This injury occurs when the astragalus and the distal end of the tibia are driven together with great violence.
When a patient falls from a height and lands on his feet, the
impact is most marked on the os calcis, astragalus and tibia.
Such injuries have been a frequent result of aircraft crash
landings.

Physical examination shows diffuse enlargement of the lower

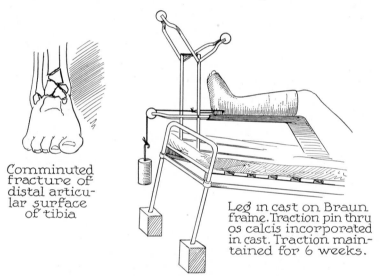

Comminuted
fracture of
distal articu-
lar surface
of tibia

Leg in cast on Braun
frame.Traction pin thru
os calcis incorporated
in cast. Traction main-
tained for 6 weeks.

FIG. 187.—Treatment of a severely comminuted fracture of the distal end
of the tibia and fibula by skeletal traction on the Braun frame.

end of the leg, broadening of the ankle, loss of normal relationship of medial and lateral malleoli, local tenderness over the
tibia, false motion and crepitus. A pressure dressing, using large
amounts of cotton or multiple gauze fluffs beneath a loose fitting
plaster cast will help minimize the swelling which may be severe
with circulatory blisters or even gangrene. Skeletal traction with
a Steinmann pin placed through the os calcis while the leg is
supported on a Braun frame may be used after the initial swell-

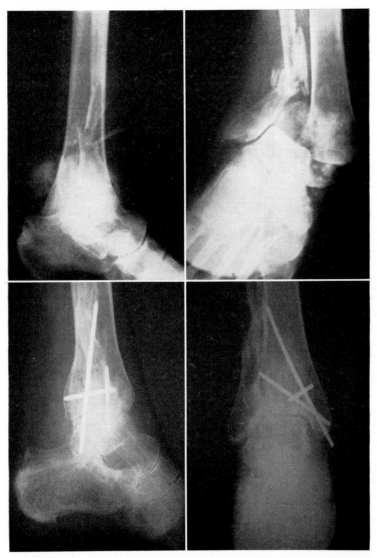

Fig. 188.—Severely comminuted, open trimalleolar fracture, treated by cleansing, débridement, fixation of reduced fragments with threaded pins, and primary closure.

345

ing subsides (Fig. 187). Severe comminution and impaction of the fragments may preclude an adequate restitution of the joint surface by traction alone. In such cases open reduction will be necessary (Fig. 188). This procedure is technically difficult and should be undertaken only by a surgeon who is highly skilled in bone surgery. Primary arthrodesis of the ankle is indicated in

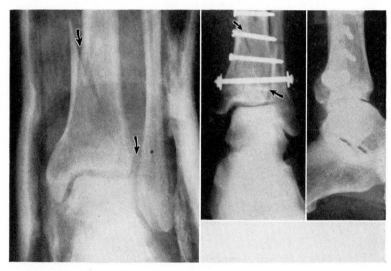

FIG. 189.—Comminuted oblique fracture of the distal tibia with separation between the tibia and fibula. It is difficult to maintain satisfactory reduction of the tibiofibular separation by closed methods. The illustration shows screw fixation of the tibial fracture with a Barr bolt through the tibia and fibula to maintain correct joint relationship.

selected cases when the derangement of the joint is severe and a painless functioning ankle cannot be expected to follow conservative management or open reduction.

DIASTASIS OF DISTAL TIBIOFIBULAR JOINT.—Separation of the distal tibiofibular joint occurs with certain abduction injuries of the ankle. Fractures of the lower third of the shaft of the fibula and of the medial malleolus frequently accompany the diastasis between the tibia and the fibula. In other instances, the malleoli remain intact and the deltoid ligament is ruptured as the tibia and fibula separate and the foot displaces laterally.

Reduction may be accomplished under general anesthesia by molding the tibia and fibula together with the foot pushed medially and in moderate varus. This position should be maintained by a short leg cast for six weeks. Open reduction with fixation of the fibula to the tibia by a long metal screw or threaded pin is advisable when closed reduction is unsuccessful (Fig. 189). Persistent diastasis with broadening of the ankle mortise will result in an unstable and painful weight-bearing joint. Arthrodesis of the ankle may be necessary to restore stability and painless function.

NONUNION OF THE MEDIAL MALLEOLUS is a common complication of fractures involving the ankle. This occurs if reduction of the original fracture is inadequate, but it is also seen in spite of excellent re-position of the fragment. A simple method of treating this nonunion has been included in this book because the technique described is not difficult and can be carried out by any competent surgeon (Fig. 190). It is well to remember, however, that this operation includes opening into the ankle joint and careless technique may lead to local infection, suppurative arthritis and a residual painful or ankylosed joint.

MALUNITED FRACTURES OF THE ANKLE.—In instances of malunion of ankle joint fractures, the end-results will include traumatic arthritis because of breakdown and roughening of articular surfaces. The treatment of choice is arthrodesis of the ankle joint. Arthrodesis is accomplished by excision of articular cartilage until bleeding bone is exposed; approximation of the astragalus to the tibia with the foot in a corrected position, and a bone graft cut from the tibia and mortised into and across the front of the joint. The foot must be placed in a position that is anatomically correct for strength and weight-bearing. In a male, the foot is immobilized for arthrodesis in 10 degrees of equinus.

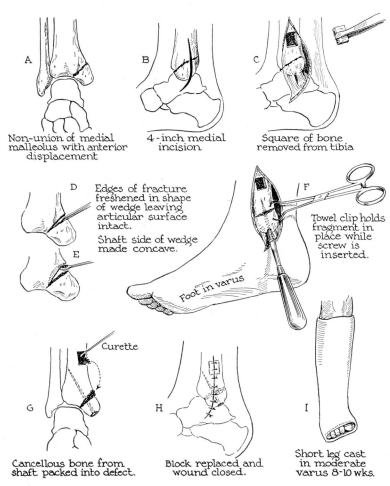

A — Non-union of medial malleolus with anterior displacement

B — 4-inch medial incision

C — Square of bone removed from tibia

D — Edges of fracture freshened in shape of wedge leaving articular surface intact.

E — Shaft side of wedge made concave.

Foot in varus

F — Towel clip holds fragment in place while screw is inserted.

G — Curette. Cancellous bone from shaft packed into defect.

H — Block replaced and wound closed.

I — Short leg cast in moderate varus 8-10 wks.

Fig. 190.—Treatment of nonunion following fracture of the medial malleolus.

348

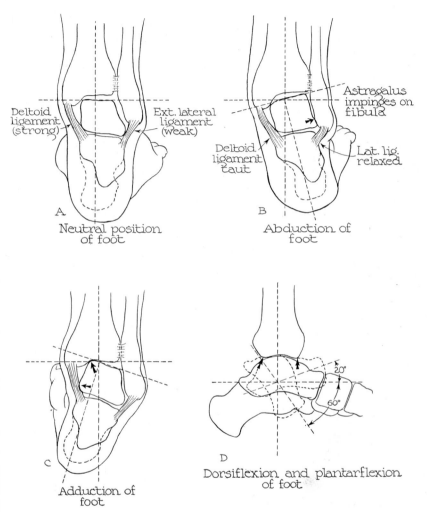

Deltoid
ligament
(strong)

Ext. lateral
ligament
(weak)

A

Neutral position
of foot

Astragalus
impinges on
fibula

Deltoid
ligament
taut

Lat. lig.
relaxed

B

Abduction of
foot

C

Adduction of
foot

20°

60°

D

Dorsiflexion and plantarflexion
of foot

FIG. 191.—Stresses and strains produced by ankle joint movement.

349

This permits full plantar surface weight-bearing in shoes with average heels. The surgeon must ascertain from a female patient the height of heels she desires to wear following surgery, and the degree of equinus should be determined accordingly. A minimum of 14 weeks is required for solid union, but weight-bearing in a short leg cast with a walking iron may be permitted after six weeks. An excellent gait is possible after ankle joint fusion if the foot has been placed in proper relationship to the tibia and the midtarsal joints are mobile.

SPRAIN.—A sprain is an injury to the ligaments. The lateral ligaments are injured most often because the range of motion and instability of the foot is greatest from the lateral toward the medial side. On the other hand, valgus motion is limited by the anatomic arrangement of the subastragalar joint and the size and tautness of the deltoid (combined medial) ligament. A relatively greater force is required to abduct the foot and injure the medial ligament as compared with the ease with which the foot may be thrown into adduction by stepping on a stone or rough pavement (Figs. 191 and 192).

The injury to the ligaments may vary from a tear of a few fibers to complete rupture or an avulsion chip fracture of the malleolus to which it is attached. The treatment and prognosis depend on an accurate evaluation of the extent of the injury.

This is best determined by roentgenograms which will also disclose the presence or absence of a fracture. If the area of tenderness is over the lateral aspect of the talus, the anterior talofibular ligament is most likely injured and an anteroposterior roentgenogram is taken with the foot in equinus and forced adduction. If this ligament alone has been ruptured, the ankle joint is less stable than normal with the foot in equinus. There is increased mobility of the subtalar joint, however, if the roentgenogram is taken with the foot at 90 degrees to the tibia.

When the tenderness is over the lateral aspect of the calcaneus, a tear of the calcaneofibular ligament is suspected and the antero-

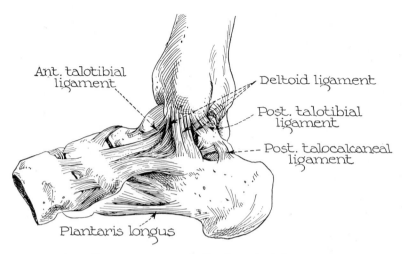

Ant. talotibial ligament

Deltoid ligament

Post. talotibial ligament

Post. talocalcaneal ligament

Plantaris longus

Medial Ligaments of Right Ankle

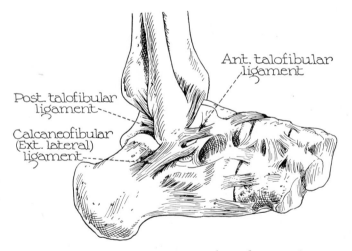

Ant. talofibular ligament

Post. talofibular ligament

Calcaneofibular (Ext. lateral) ligament

Lateral Ligaments of Right Ankle

Fig. 192.—The supporting ligaments of the ankle joint.

351

posterior roentgenogram is taken with the foot in forced varus and the talus at 90 degrees with the tibia. There is increased

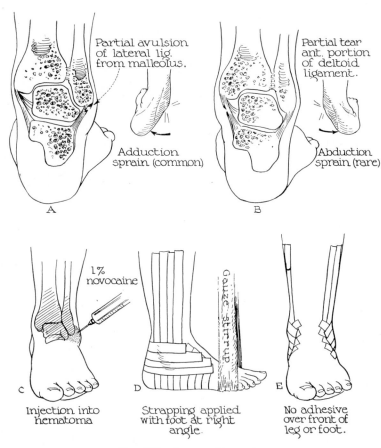

Partial avulsion of lateral lig. from malleolus.

Adduction sprain (common)

Partial tear ant. portion of deltoid ligament.

Abduction sprain (rare)

A

B

1% novocaine

Gauze stirrup

C   D   E

Injection into hematoma

Strapping applied with foot at right angle.

No adhesive over front of leg or foot.

FIG. 193.—Acute ankle sprains.

motion in the subtalar joint and a slight increase in the ankle joint if the ligament is torn. The talotibial joint is essentially stable if the roentgenogram is taken with the foot in equinus.

When both the calcaneofibular and anterior talofibular ligaments are ruptured, the ankle and subtalar joints are unstable with the foot at either 90 degrees or in equinus. The talus will move out of the mortise of the tibia and fibula and leave a gap between the tibia and the talus on the side of the torn ligaments.

Minor sprains may be associated with outstanding pain, disability and swelling caused by hemorrhage. The patient may have meager symptoms for 30 minutes to several hours after the injury, after which the pain becomes severe and walking on the foot is impossible. Minor sprains may be treated by the local infiltration of 5 to 10 cc. of 1 per cent procaine into the tender areas and the application of an adhesive tape splint (Fig. 193). Crutches should be used only if severe pain prevents the patient from bearing full weight on the extremity. The adhesive strapping should be worn from seven to 14 days. If the patient is co-operative and continues to be active with weight-bearing, there will be little swelling after this splinting is discontinued. One-quarter inch heel elevation on the side of the ligament injury will give the patient a feeling of security and guard against mild trauma and pain associated with walking on uneven ground.

Complete rupture of an ankle joint ligament should be treated by six weeks of plaster of paris cast immobilization (Fig. 194). The patient may bear weight in the cast. A heel wedge of 3/16 to 1/4 in. offers further protection to the healing ligaments after the cast is discarded. A chronic, recurrent sprain of the ankle may be the late manifestation of an acute rupture which was not properly diagnosed or adequately treated and may require surgical repair of the injured ligament. Others are caused by internal derangement of the ankle joint in which a projection of tissue becomes caught between the astragalus and the lateral malleolus. The treatment consists of excision of the offending tissue.

In OPEN FRACTURES OR IN FRACTURE-DISLOCATIONS of the ankle, the wound must be carefully excised, the joint irrigated with warm normal saline solution, the capsule closed and the skin sutured loosely, if conditions permit (see Chapter XI). One

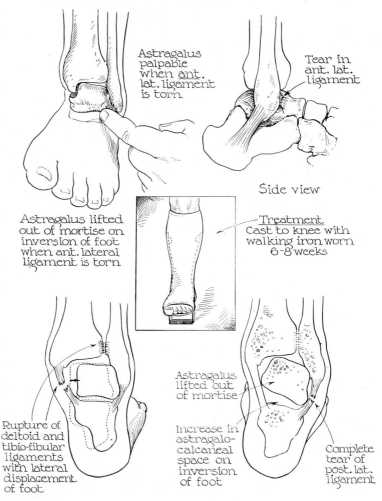

Astragalus palpable when ant. lat. ligament is torn

Tear in ant. lat. ligament

Side view

Astragalus lifted out of mortise on inversion of foot when ant. lateral ligament is torn

Treatment
Cast to knee with walking iron worn 6-8 weeks

Rupture of deltoid and tibio-fibular ligaments with lateral displacement of foot

Astragalus lifted out of mortise

Increase in astragalo-calcaneal space on inversion of foot

Complete tear of post. lat. ligament

FIG. 194.—Tear of ligaments of the ankle with subluxation of the astragalus or the foot.

354

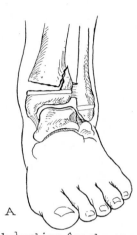

A

Abduction fracture with
epiphyseal dislocation of
tibia. Not likely to result
in growth disturbance.

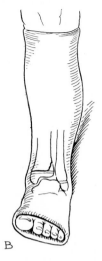

B

Put up in short
leg cast with
foot in moderate
adduction.

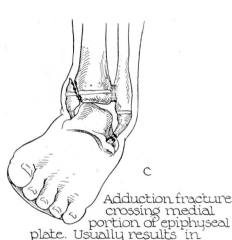

C

Adduction fracture
crossing medial
portion of epiphyseal
plate. Usually results in
growth disturbance.

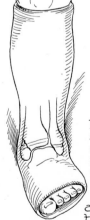

D

Put up in
short leg
cast with
foot in
abduction.
Reduction
force
accomplished
thru untorn
medial ligament and
molding of fragment.

Fig. 195.—Fractures of distal end of the growing tibia.

should not hesitate to use screws or pins to control the position of the fragments. The subsequent treatment should be by plaster cast immobilization in a position which will maintain the reduction.

INJURIES OF THE GROWTH CARTILAGE.—The automobile, the bicycle and competitive sports all contribute to the problem of injuries of the growth cartilages of children. With the exception of the elbow and wrist, the ankle is the most common site of

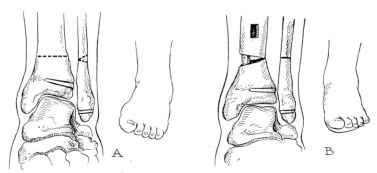

Closure of medial third of plate with continued growth of lateral portion. Progressive adduction deformity.

Slight overcorrection by repeated supramalleolar osteotomy until epiphyseal plate completely closes.

FIG. 196.—Osteotomy for correction of adduction deformity following partial growth arrest of the tibia, the result of a fracture which caused a bone bridge to form across the epiphyseal growth cartilage.

epiphyseal fractures or traumatic displacements. Following a fracture that includes the growth cartilage zone at the distal end of the tibia as well as a portion of the shaft, regardless of how accurate the reduction, growth disturbance may follow (Fig. 195). Growth arrest of a portion of the distal epiphyseal cartilage may produce a marked varus or valgus deformity, depending on which portion of the epiphyseal plate is involved.

Treatment of the deformity caused by such premature fusion of the tibial epiphysis may include osteotomy (Fig. 196), fol-

lowed by an operation to arrest growth completely in the portion
of the epiphyseal cartilage which is still functioning. This surgical
arrest of growth is accomplished by excising a segment of the
epiphyseal cartilage and bridging between the epiphysis and the
metaphysis with a tibial bone graft. Growth of the distal end of
the fibula must be arrested at the same time. When this operation is carried out on one leg, inequality of leg length may be
prevented or minimized by performing epiphyseodesis of the
opposite distal tibial and fibular epiphyses.

CHAPTER XXIX

The Foot

DISABILITY resulting from fractures, sprains or dislocations of the foot is often far in excess of what one might expect from studying the initial injury. Loss of motion between the midtarsal joints or the tarsal-metatarsal joints as a result of adhesions which form after any of the aforementioned injuries may produce so much pain and disability that the patient becomes a chronic invalid. Presence of adhesions in the foot is not uncommon after major injuries to other regions of the limb which require long immobilization of the foot as a part of the treatment. Following any long period of plaster cast immobilization there is circulatory edema after the cast has been removed. Much of the disability associated with cast immobilization, or that following a specific injury to the foot, can be prevented by co-operation between patient and surgeon. The use of a walking iron, the molding of the cast beneath the weight-bearing surface of the foot, so that support is given to both the metatarsal and the longitudinal arch, and early active motion will greatly reduce the incidence of serious disability.

FRACTURE OF THE OS CALCIS.—This is the most challenging of all the problems of injury to single bones of the foot. No fracture, with the exception of that of the neck of the femur, has yielded more consistently unsatisfactory results in the hands of the average surgeon. It should be remembered that every fracture of the os calcis which results from a fall from a height is likely to be associated with an injury to the spine (Fig. 197) and should routinely call for examination and possibly roentgen study of the other foot and of the spine. In direct weight-bearing

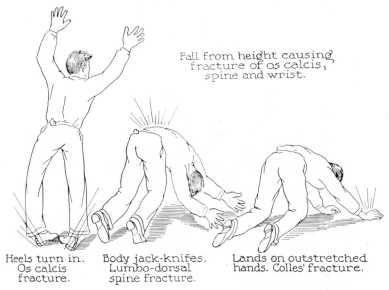

Fall from height causing fracture of os calcis, spine and wrist.

Heels turn in. Os calcis fracture.

Body jack-knifes. Lumbo-dorsal spine fracture.

Lands on outstretched hands. Colles' fracture.

FIG. 197.—Mechanism of production of os calcis fractures and commonly associated injuries.

line, the tibia articulates with the astragalus and the astragalus with the os calcis. In severe crushing fractures, the astragalus may be driven completely through the os calcis to occupy a position inferior to it on the plantar surface of the foot (Fig. 198). Impacted fractures of the os calcis may be overlooked in the initial examination.

A comprehensive study of the os calcis fractures in which they were classified with regard to the different types was made by

Vidal and adopted by Boehler. The three significant groups are:
(1) isolated fracture without joint injury; (2) comminuted fracture with minimal joint injury, such as a crack through the body

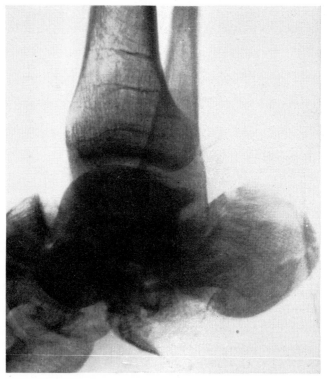

Fig. 198.—A third degree fracture of the os calcis. The astragalus has been
driven down between the fragments. Prognosis for a satisfactory functional
recovery is not good.

without displacement, or fracture of the outer wall and the body,
with a reduction of the tuber-joint angle but no crushing into
the joint, and (3) comminuted fracture with severe joint injury,
with reduced tuber-joint angle and displacement or crushing of
portions of the body. From the standpoint of treatment, each of

these three types of fracture necessitates special consideration.
The problem in general, however, is to restore the tuber-joint

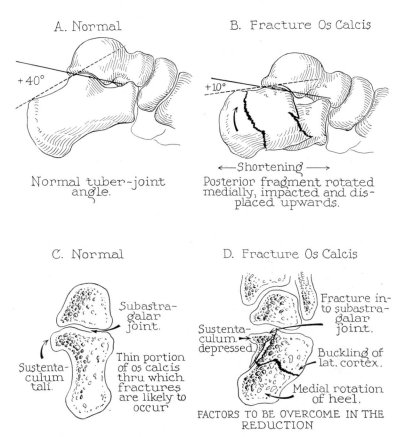

A. Normal

+40°

Normal tuber-joint
angle.

B. Fracture Os Calcis

+10°

←— Shortening —→
Posterior fragment rotated
medially, impacted and displaced upwards.

C. Normal

Subastra-
galar
joint.

Sustenta-
culum
tali.

Thin portion
of os calcis
thru which
fractures
are likely to
occur

D. Fracture Os Calcis

Fracture in-
to subastra-
galar
joint.

Sustenta-
culum
depressed.

Buckling of
lat. cortex.

Medial rotation
of heel.

FACTORS TO BE OVERCOME IN THE
REDUCTION

Fig. 199.—Fracture of the os calcis with inversion deformity and decrease
in the tuber-joint angle.

angle, reduce the transverse diameter approximately to normal
and replace the joint surfaces as accurately as possible. It is impossible to diagnose, plan or carry out treatment intelligently
and accurately without having roentgenograms that are made in

the anteroposterior, lateral and axial planes. By axial plane we mean a roentgenogram made plantar-dorsally and showing the relationship of the astragalus or astragalar fragments to the intermalleolar borders. The tuber-joint angle of the os calcis is important and should be restored if possible (Fig. 199). It is an angle between a line projected backward from the anterior and posterior articular surfaces and the line of the upper margin of the tuberosity. Normally it measures 35–45 degrees. Following

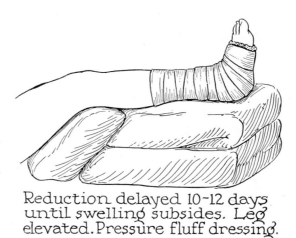

Reduction delayed 10-12 days until swelling subsides. Leg elevated. Pressure fluff dressing.

Fig. 200.—Elastic bandage pressure dressing to help reduce swelling that follows fracture of the os calcis.

a severe fracture it may be reduced to 5 or 10 degrees or obliterated altogether. Occasionally it is even reversed. This disturbance of the tuber-joint angle weakens or seriously interferes with the action of the gastrocnemius muscle.

Treatment.—Correction of fractures of the os calcis requires skill and experience. Time of the reduction depends to a considerable extent on how soon after the injury the patient is seen by the fracture surgeon. If swelling has not yet become excessive, the fracture may be reduced at once. Should the patient be delayed in reaching the hospital and swelling is excessive, a massive pressure dressing should be applied from the toes to the knee, the limb elevated, the foot of the bed raised and attempts at reduction deferred until swelling subsides (Fig. 200).

Fractures of the os calcis without loss of the tuber-joint angle or spread of the os calcis or extensive comminution of an articular surface may be treated without any attempt at reduction

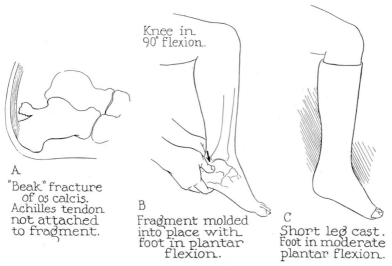

Fig. 201.—Minimal fracture of the tuber portion of the os calcis.

(Fig. 201). A plaster cast should be applied, extending from just back of the toes to the tibial tubercle. A walking iron should be placed in the cast and the patient encouraged to bear sufficient weight to balance himself, but not to attempt any walking without crutches for six weeks. At the end of this time the cast is removed and an elastic bandage is applied to prevent excessive edema. The patient should then continue with crutches while gradually increasing weight-bearing.

If the fracture includes a spread of the os calcis without loss of tuber-joint angle, a redresser should be applied and the os calcis firmly compressed from side to side. The C-shaped redresser should be placed beneath the lateral malleolus. (It is wise to test the normal foot first, to determine the thickness of the normal os calcis, together with the soft tissue covering.) The clamp is rapidly closed to the mark on the measuring device which corresponds to that of the normal heel, then rapidly opened. If pressure is continued for more than one or two minutes at the most, necrosis of the tissues may result. It is not necessary to place a thick felt pad over the os calcis if the procedure is performed swiftly and skilfully.

Horizontal incomplete fractures of the proximal third of the tuber portion of the os calcis are called "beak" fractures (Fig. 201). The fragment can usually be molded downward into place and a short leg cast is applied for six weeks. When manual re-position is unsuccessful, a Steinmann pin may be passed transversely through the soft tissues above the fragment and downward traction will usually reduce the angulated fragment.

Another infrequent but distinctly different fracture of the os calcis consists of a vertical break in its tuber portion with the posterior fragment pulled upward by the gastrocnemius and soleus muscles (Fig. 202). Reduction is readily accomplished by a single Steinmann pin which is used as a lever and then incorporated in the short leg cast to prevent re-displacement of the fragment. Union is sufficiently advanced at six weeks to allow partial weight-bearing with crutches for an additional four weeks. Care must be exercised to avoid pressure necrosis of the soft tissues by the pin. This predisposes to infection along the pin tract which is a most unfortunate complication for the patient.

Accurate reduction of comminuted fractures of the os calcis, with excessive upward displacement of the tuber fragment, broadening of the body and minimal involvement of the joint surfaces, is most readily accomplished by means of skeletal traction and fixation. A Boehler os calcis frame (Fig. 203), or one of the newer type of fracture tables, may be used. In the Boehler method the thigh is flexed 45–50 degrees and the knee at least 45 degrees, with a padded bar or strong sling supporting the leg just above the knee. A Steinmann pin is then placed through the os calcis near the site of insertion of the Achilles tendon. Traction

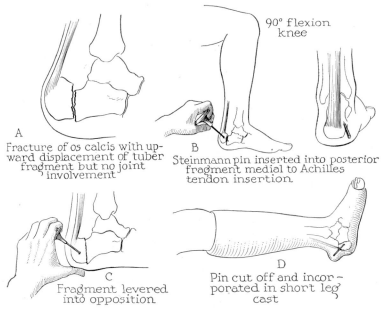

A
Fracture of os calcis with upward displacement of tuber
fragment but no joint
involvement

B
Steinmann pin inserted into posterior
fragment medial to Achilles
tendon insertion.

90° flexion
knee

C
Fragment levered
into opposition.

D
Pin cut off and incor-
porated in short leg
cast

Fig. 202.—Single pin method of reduction and immobilization of vertical fractures of the tuber portion of the os calcis.

is applied directly in line with the tibia by a turnbuckle or the ratchet apparatus of the fracture table. This traction must be sufficient to restore the tuber-joint angle. When it is apparent that this angle has been restored, the direction of pull is shifted down and back to obtain lengthening of the os calcis (Fig. 204). While traction is maintained in the direction of the second pull described, another Steinmann pin is drilled, either through the

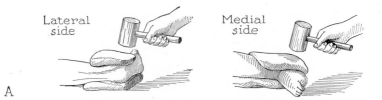

Lateral
side

Medial
side

A

Buckling of cortex corrected by hitting padded heel with mallet.

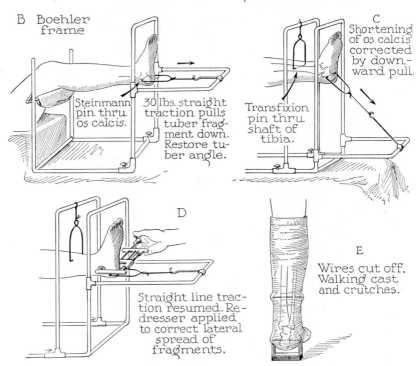

B Boehler
frame

Steinmann pin thru os calcis. 30 lbs. straight traction pulls tuber fragment down. Restore tuber angle.

C Shortening of os calcis corrected by downward pull.

Transfixion pin thru shaft of tibia.

D

Straight line traction resumed. Redresser applied to correct lateral spread of fragments.

E

Wires cut off. Walking cast and crutches.

FIG. 203.—Reduction of the comminuted os calcis fracture. Ambulation with crutches is permitted at once, but no weight-bearing for six weeks.

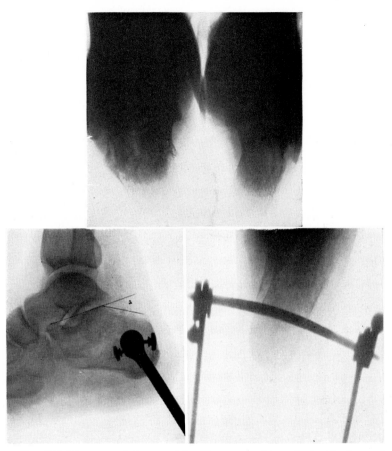

Fig. 204.—Fracture of the os calcis. *Above,* note the marked widening and shortening of the neck portion. *Below left,* restoration of the tuber-joint angle by skeletal traction. *Below right,* restoration of length after molding the comminuted fragments beneath the malleoli with a Boehler redresser.

367

lower shaft of the tibia 3 in. above the ankle joint or through
the tibia just below the tuberosity. A Boehler re-dresser is then
applied, as recommended in the preceding section, and the
widening of the os calcis rapidly corrected by tightening the
clamp.

A cast is applied while traction is maintained, and both pins
are incorporated in the plaster. The cast is carefully molded over
firm rolls of felt placed below the malleoli. The transfixion pins
should not be removed for six weeks, during which time the
patient may be ambulatory on crutches. Roentgenograms should
be made after reduction and again within one week after the
cast is applied. At the end of six weeks the pins and cast are
removed. Roentgenograms should be made and a new cast applied, incorporating a walking iron. Weight-bearing may then
be permitted. When the second cast is removed, 12 weeks after
the first reduction, an elastic bandage should be applied to control or prevent excessive edema. If the patient is moderately
active during the period while immobilization is being maintained, first by the pins and cast, and later by the cast alone,
there will be comparatively little atrophy of disuse, and the
patient may be able to return to work within five months of the
time of the injury.

Fractures of the os calcis which disrupt the articular surface
for the subtalar joint carry the least favorable prognosis of this
group of injuries. They are ordinarily associated with broadening of the tuber portion of the os calcis and a decrease in the
tuber joint angle. Two types of fractures of the joint surface are
frequently encountered. In one the articular cartilage and varying sized fragments of bone are rotated downward and forward
as much as 90 degrees so as to be impacted into the adjacent
cancellous bone (Fig. 205). The second type consists of a horizontal fracture along the superior aspect of the os calcis which
extends forward to emerge anteriorly and distally to the subtalar
joint. The articular end of the fragment is rotated downward so

that the joint surface faces in the direction of the toes, while the other end is displaced upward. This results in a V-shaped defect similar to a "beak" fracture, except that it is longer and contains

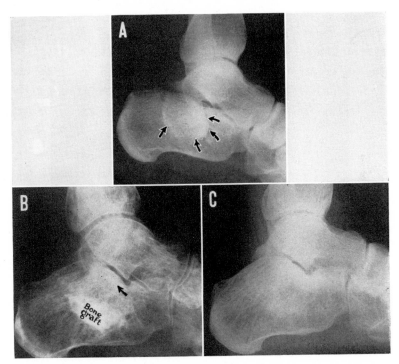

Fig. 205.—Fracture of the os calcis with loss of the tuber joint angle and marked depression and rotation of the calcaneal joint surface, *A*. Treated surgically by restoration of the articular surface and the use of bone grafts packed snugly beneath the elevated fragment, *B*. For comparison, *C* illustrates the normal opposite subtalar joint.

varying sized portions of the articular cartilage. There is no way to restore the contour of the os calcis and to reconstruct the subtalar joint except by open reduction.

For open reduction or subtalar fusion, an incision begins behind the fibula, 3 in. above the lateral malleolus, and extends distally over the lateral aspect of the os calcis to end at the calcaneocuboid joint. The peroneus longus and brevis tendons are mobilized and retracted after cutting their tendon sheaths and the superior and inferior peroneal retinaculum. The calcaneofibular ligament and the trochlear process of the os calcis are exposed in the wound. The lateral broadening of the os calcis in comminuted fractures is in part due to a fracture and separa-

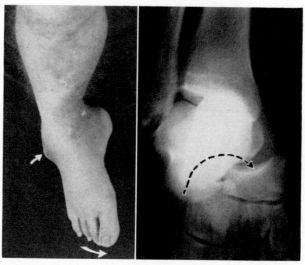

Fig. 206.—A medial subtalar and talonavicular dislocation. Reduction frequently requires strong skeletal traction or, occasionally, an open reduction.

tion of the trochlear process and the adjacent cortex. This fragment is retracted laterally and the subtalar joint is exposed as a linear incision is made in the calcaneofibular ligament. The impacted fragment is elevated by means of a chisel and the articular surface replaced accurately. A moderate sized defect remains in the os calcis below the elevated fragment and is filled by means of a bone graft from the tibia or ilium (Fig. 205, B). The graft holds the articular fragment in position. The wound is closed in layers and a short leg cast is worn for three months.

Late disabling arthritis often results following this procedure. Therefore a primary subtalar arthrodesis is recommended for these severe fractures which merit open reduction. The technique consists of restoration of the fragments as described, and removal of the articular cartilage from the talus and calcaneus. Cancellous and cortical bone chips should be packed into the joint space.

FRACTURES OF THE ASTRAGALUS.—Fractures of the posterior tubercle or the neck of the astragalus may be isolated or may accompany fractures of the os calcis. Fractures of the posterior tubercle may produce few symptoms. Occasionally, a separation of this posterior portion of the bone is found in both feet, suggesting that this may be due to a congenital anomaly in which the tubercle develops as a separate ossicle. The astragalus is sometimes crushed and driven down completely into or through fragments of a fractured os calcis (Fig. 198). Aseptic necrosis of the body of the astragalus may occur when fracture of the neck also disrupts the anterior nutrient artery. A severe crushing fracture of the astragalus, with dislocation, is best treated by complete excision of this bone. Fractures of the neck only can be treated by manipulation; usually it is not difficult to restore the anatomic position of the fragments. A plaster cast with a walking iron should then be worn for eight to 10 weeks.

FRACTURES OF THE MIDTARSAL BONES OF THE FOOT.—These bones consist of the cuboid, scaphoid and three cuneiforms. A fracture should be reduced as accurately as possible by manipulation under complete anesthesia. The arch and normal contour of the foot are molded and a plaster cast dressing is applied (Fig. 207). Weight-bearing should be permitted after the second, or at latest the third week.

Injuries with or without roentgenographically demonstrable fracture of the scaphoid bone are sometimes followed by complete disintegration of the bone, due to aseptic necrosis. This is usually spoken of as Koehler's disease. When it is present, the

foot should be protected from weight-bearing. A plaster boot
should be worn until the roentgenograms show marked improvement in the appearance of this bone.

Fractures of any one or of all of the five metatarsal bones may
be either transverse or oblique. They may occur in the cancellous
region of the distal ends of these bones as a result of the strain
during walking. Fractures of the shafts of the metatarsals are
sometimes followed by over-riding, and a combination fracture

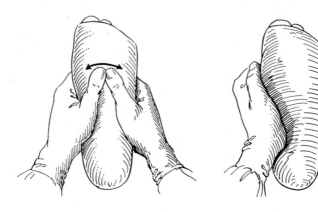

Molding up transverse   Molding longi-
arch on plantar surface   tudinal arch of
of foot cast.   foot cast.

Fig. 207.—The cast should be molded to support the foot.

of the shaft with dislocation of the metatarsal-phalangeal joint
is exceedingly difficult to treat effectively. The metatarsal bones
must be restored to length. If there is over-riding, there is no
way of obtaining an effective grasp of the bone by ordinary
casts or splints. Such fractures produce serious disability if they
are not recognized and reduced and the reduction maintained
until healing takes place.

Reduction of fractures with displacement or of fracture-
dislocations of the metatarsals and metatarsal-phalangeal joints

is best obtained by traction (Fig. 208). Short pieces of Kirschner wires or special wire clips are introduced through the tough tissue at the distal ends of the toes of the respective fractured or dislocated metatarsal bones. Attachment of traction to the toe-nails is painful and should not be used. A plaster cast from the tibial tubercle downward to include the metatarsal region is

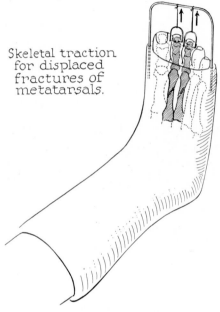

Skeletal traction for displaced fractures of metatarsals.

FIG. 208.—Oblique or over-riding fractures of the metatarsals.

then applied. A wire loop made from an old coat hanger is in-corporated in the cast in such a way that it extends about 3 in. beyond the ends of the toes. Rubber bands are then applied to produce continuous traction on the toes (Fig. 209). In fracture-dislocation, it may be necessary to do an open operation or to introduce a steel pin to fix the distal fracture fragment of the metatarsal while traction is made on the toe to reduce the

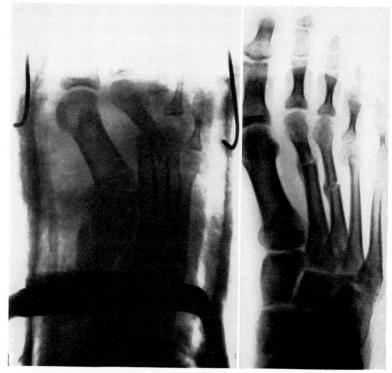

Fig. 209.—Fracture-dislocation of the metatarsal bones of the foot are best treated by continuous rubber band traction.

metatarsal-phalangeal articulation. This traction is maintained for three weeks, at the end of which time the traction wires may be removed. The patient continues to use a plaster cast with a walking iron for a further period of three weeks.

FRACTURES OF THE PHALANGES of the toes without displacement rarely require definitive treatment. Splinting to adjacent uninjured toes usually suffices. If there is displacement with overriding, continuous traction, as already described, should be used.

PART IV

Fractures and Dislocations of the Trunk

CHAPTER XXX

The Spine

THE compression fracture of the spine, known as the jackknife fracture, is produced by an injury which doubles the body up into a position of extreme flexion. The vertebral body is crushed and wedged until it is more narrow anteriorly than it is in its posterior portion (Fig. 210). Occasionally, a direct fall onto the buttocks or pressure from a weight coming directly on the shoulders, with the spine extended, produces a central compression of one or more vertebral bodies. Severe trauma, such as that which may be incurred in an automobile accident or a train wreck, may include multiple fractures of the spine, with injuries to many transverse processes, fractures of pedicles and laminae, injury of the vertebral bodies and, occasionally, dislocation. Such injuries are nearly always attended by some damage to the spinal cord or the nerve roots, or both. There may be a complete transection of the cord, with permanent paralysis below the level of transection.

VERTEBRAL BODIES.—Simple compression fractures should be reduced. If the fracture consists merely of wedging, without a marked spread or increase in the anteroposterior diameter of the bone, a satisfactory reduction can be obtained in most instances by forced hyperextension. Fortunately, this type of fracture represents about 60 per cent of the vertebral body injuries. Hyperextension can accomplish appreciable reduction because to the anterior and lateral borders of both superior and inferior margins

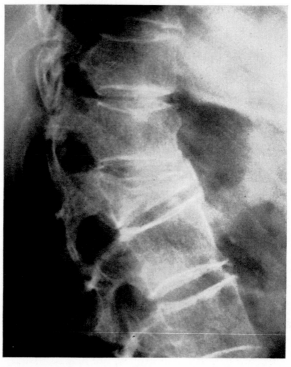

Fig. 210.—Unreduced fracture of thoracic vertebra. The injury had been incurred four years previously and was not recognized.

of each vertebral body are attached the powerful vertical fibers of the annulus fibrosis. When the spine is hyperextended, these fibers become taut and pull the bone fragments back into position. Even in cases with badly comminuted fractures, a considerable amount of improvement in position will result from hyperextension. If the fracture is central, with crushing in of the articular plate over the central portion of the weight-bearing surface of the vertebral bodies, no reduction can be anticipated because there are no strong fibrous attachments between the vertebral bodies centrally. This area of the bone is in contact with the nucleus pulposus of the intervertebral disk and is covered by a layer of hyaline cartilage.

HYPEREXTENSION OF COMPRESSION FRACTURES

Apparatus for obtaining reduction of compression type fractures have varied from an automobile jack to exceedingly complicated appliances provided by manufacturers of orthopedic fracture tables. The *Watson-Jones method* is the simplest and probably the most efficient. According to this procedure, the patient is placed face down upon two tables in such a way that the tables come together underneath the abdomen at the level of the fractured vertebral body. The tables are slowly drawn apart until only the patient's legs, to the midthigh, rest on one table, while the arms and chin rest on the other (Fig. 211). An assistant must hold the arms securely in position while a second assistant protects or holds the legs. The weight of the patient produces hyperextension of the spine as the body sags between the two tables. The surgeon then places the heel of his palm against the most prominent spinous process and, by gentle pressure and kneading, reduces this process until it is no longer prominent. A plaster cast is then applied, reaching to the sternal notch in front above and to the symphysis below. The cast should be padded with a thin layer of felt over the posterior spinous processes and the crests of the ilium and the sternum. The cast can be more neatly trimmed if stockinette is pulled over the trunk before reduction is started.

The *Davis method* is also quite satisfactory. The patient is placed face down on a canvas sling 6 in. wide, and the feet are gradually elevated to obtain the desired overextension of the spine. After the cast is applied, following reduction of the fracture, the patient may be ambulatory within two days and is encouraged to be as active as possible.

Inadequate reduction and completely ineffective casts are the two outstanding causes of the poor results so often seen in these cases. To obtain good immobilization, the cast must extend so high and so low in front that it cannot afford any real comfort, and the patient will invariably object to it. He should be told in

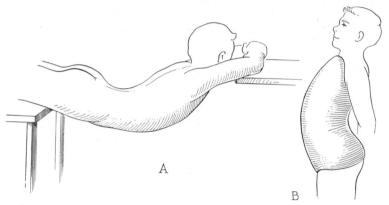

Fig. 211.—Simple method of reduction of a compression fracture of the spine and application of the hyperextension jacket.

advance, and may have to be reminded again and again, that the purpose of the cast is to splint his broken back rather than to make him comfortable. Unless the patient is willing to endure some inconvenience and discomfort, a poor result may be expected. As a rule, patients are not able to return to active work for six to 10 months after fractures of the spine.

Fractures of the transverse or posterior spinous processes require no treatment other than rest in bed for 10 to 14 days until the acute soreness in the muscles subsides.

Fracture-dislocation without spinal cord injury is an indication for spinal fusion, after obtaining as good a reduction as possible.

In acute fractures with evidence of spinal cord involvement, an attempt should be made to determine whether there is complete transection, as evidenced by total paralysis below the level of the fracture. If the paralysis is only partial, the conservative course is to wait several days to see whether recovery takes place. If paralysis is total, the spinal cord either has been divided or is being compressed by a fragment of bone, or there is extensive hemorrhage into the spinal cord. A laminectomy is of little value unless performed immediately. It is indicated if on spinal puncture the Queckenstedt test shows total block of the subarachnoid space.

Old compression fractures of the spine cannot be changed by manipulation. If a lame back persists, an operation to produce arthrodesis, using a tibial bone graft, is recommended.

Occasionally fractures of the spine are produced by hyperextension. The injury is most often localized to the posterior appendages of the spine, such as the laminae, articular facets or posterior spinous processes. A body cast without hyperextension is indicated.

FRACTURES AND DISLOCATIONS OF THE CERVICAL SPINE.— Formerly, these occurred most often as a result of diving into shallow water. Mechanized warfare and training of large numbers of men as parachute jumpers have increased the incidence of fracture-dislocations of the neck vertebrae. Simple compression fractures may be reduced by hyperextension and traction. The patient is placed on his back on an ordinary operating table or fracture table and is drawn well out over the end of the table with his head and neck supported, by an assistant, in a position of hyperextension. Each of the new fracture tables has a special arrangement for obtaining traction and hyperextension of the cervical spine, while supporting the body in a position which permits application of a cast.

Fracture combined with dislocation of both articular facets at the same level is frequently associated with such severe injury to the spinal cord that paralysis occurs within three or four hours after the injury. If the injury is in the upper cervical region, death is almost certain. Immobilization of fractures with unilateral or bilateral dislocation is accomplished most effectively by a plaster cast which holds the head securely in position of hyperextension and extends down on the body to the level of

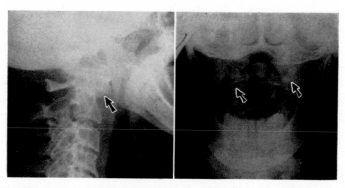

FIG. 212.—Fracture-dislocation between first and second cervical vertebrae. The odontoid process is fractured at its base and there is a fracture with displacement in the left lateral articular process of the first cervical vertebra. Strong, carefully controlled, skeletal tong traction is required for reduction and maintenance of position.

the umbilicus or as far as the crests of the ileum for fractures of the lower cervical spine.

Few injuries are more difficult to treat or are attended by greater danger to the life of the patient than those of fracture-dislocation in the cervical spine. Recommendations are often made for reduction of these dislocations by manipulation under anesthesia, but the danger of transection of the spinal cord as a result of such manipulations is sufficient to make even the most courageous surgeon hesitate. Strong and continuous traction will often succeed where forced manipulation has failed (Fig. 212). Occasionally it may be necessary to remove a portion of the

inferior articular facet to reduce the superior facet which has
been displaced forward. Traction may be obtained by a head
halter. If this method of traction is continued for several days,
the chin or the occiput may become exceedingly swollen, or
actual pressure necrosis may result. Skeletal traction, preferably
with calipers which attach to the calvarium through double burr

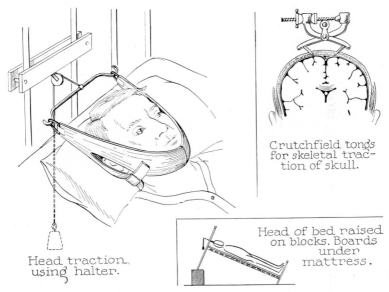

Crutchfield tongs
for skeletal trac-
tion of skull.

Head traction
using halter.

Head of bed raised
on blocks. Boards
under
mattress.

Fig. 213.—Skeletal traction is more efficient and is better tolerated by
the patient.

holes, is far more comfortable and also more efficient in obtaining and maintaining a reduction (Fig. 213). When reduction
has been obtained through skeletal traction, application of the
cast is less difficult since there is no interference from traction
equipment and no danger of losing position. The cast should
be carefully molded to chin and occiput, back of the neck,
shoulders and trunk (Fig. 214).

In general, the higher the fracture or the dislocation in the cervical spine, the greater the incidence of injury to the spinal cord. More fractures of the cervical spine occur at about the level of the fourth to the sixth vertebral bodies than at any other level. Occasionally, fractures of the atlas, with or without dis-

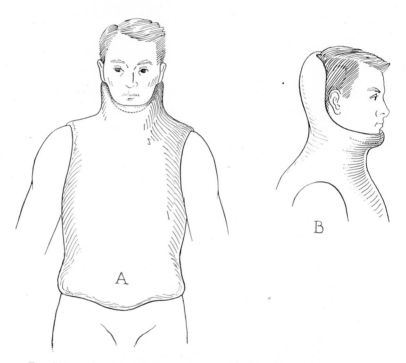

Fig. 214.—Cast immobilization of the cervical or upper thoracic spine.

location, result from a fall on the head. Cord lesions occur in approximately 50 per cent of these cases. Skeletal traction is recommended for two weeks or longer if paraplegia persists.

After six weeks to three months the plaster cast for immobilizing the cervical spine, following dislocation or fracture, may be removed and a lighter cervical spine splint may be worn for the remainder of the period for which protection and support are planned (Fig. 215). For this purpose we use a light weight plaster splint made of Johnson & Johnson ready-prepared 5 in. wide "specialists' splints." As the plaster is applied directly to

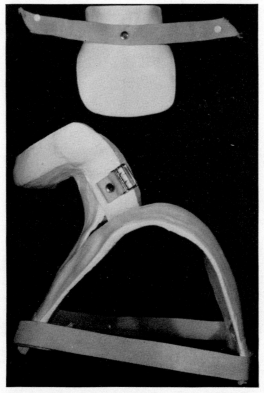

FIG. 215.—Side view of waterproofed plaster splint for the cervical spine.

the patient's skin and is molded to the contour of the neck and shoulders, an accurate fit is assured, and this means a comfortable splint. The total cost of materials does not exceed $4.00, and the delay between ordering and delivering the collar to the patient need not be more than 30 hours (Fig. 216).

BUILDING THE CERVICAL PLASTER SPLINT

Measurements are taken of the approximate lengths of the chin support, the shoulder strips, the front and back crosspieces which connect the extremities of the shoulder strips and the two struts on each side which anchor the chinpiece to the chest portion. The pieces for the chin support are made by folding over

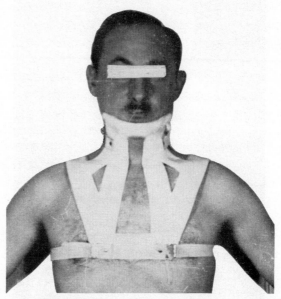

Fig. 216.—Cervical spine brace made of pre-prepared specialist's splints. It is comfortable, removable, inexpensive and waterproof and affords satisfactory immobilization.

one third of the width of the "specialist splint" lengthwise so that it is approximately 3½ in. instead of 5 in. wide. This also re-enforces one margin, which is placed in front of the chin. All other strips are made by folding the splint lengthwise twice, so that each is three layers thick and one-third the original width. Enough strips are folded so that the final thickness of each part of the collar will be made up of six such folded strips.

The patient is seated on a stool with an assistant holding the head in the desired position. A thin layer of petrolatum is smeared over the chin, neck and thorax to prevent the plaster from adhering to the skin and hairs. Two thicknesses of plaster for the chin support are first applied, making sure that there are no wrinkles and that an adequate platform has been provided beneath the chin for support of the head. Two thicknesses of shoulder strips are then applied on each side, and their front and back extremities are connected by crosspieces. The shoulder pieces must be placed sufficiently wide apart over the scapulae so that the collar can be readily removed over the head. Now the two oblique struts are placed on each side. The front struts extend from the top margin of the chinpiece at the angles of the jaw to the anterior extremities of the shoulder strips. The posterior strips join the shoulder pieces just in front of the points at which they cross the clavicles. This pattern, while affording strength where there is stress and strain, permits ventilation on all sides, a fact much appreciated during warm weather, and at the same time reduces the weight of the collar.

After the initial outline of the dressing has been completed, each strip is re-enforced until the desired thickness is obtained.

While the plaster is setting on the patient, the restraining pad for the back of the neck can be made. Ten to 12 thicknesses of 5 in. splints cut to the desired length are molded to the contour of the posterior surface of the head, neck and shoulders. In some cases a strap of 1 in. webbing over a felt pad across the back of the neck is sufficient to prevent the patient from lifting his chin out of the collar.

When the plaster has become sufficiently hardened, the collar is carefully removed and placed under a lamp or on a radiator for rapid drying. The margins are trimmed and sandpapered so that no rough or pointed edges are present to irritate the skin.

To give additional strength to the collar and at the same time make it waterproof and prevent undue soiling, five coats of the following mixture are applied to the plaster:

Sufficient acetone is added to ¾ gal. of cellulose-acetate to make 1 gal. of mixture; to this, 6 oz. of dimethyl phthalate is added and sufficient titanium dioxide to impart a white color.

Finally, 1 in. straps and buckles are applied (Figs. 215 and 216). Ordinarily soft padding is not required for the chin or shoulders if the collar conforms smoothly to the contours of the part and the head was held in a comfortable position during building of the collar.

CHAPTER XXXI

The Pelvis

FRACTURES of the pelvis occur as a result of direct violence. They are occasionally associated with injuries which result from automobile accidents or from falls from considerable heights, with the individual striking on the lower part of the back. Fractures of the sacrum are much less common than are those of the iliac, pubic or ischial bones. A crushing injury sometimes results in multiple fractures with separation of the pubic bones at the symphysis and of the sacroiliac articulations. There may be associated injuries to the urethra or bladder and paralysis of some of the sacral nerves, with loss of urinary control and sexual power. Local pain and inability to stand or walk are outstanding symptoms.

Fractures of the ilium or of a pubic or ischial ramus, without any displacement, may be treated by adhesive strapping and rest in bed; they will heal within three to six weeks. If the fracture is unilateral, the patient may begin walking, using crutches and bearing weight on the leg of the uninjured side, within three weeks after the injury occurs, but at least six weeks should elapse before weight is borne on the side of the fracture.

Fractures of the ilium, ischium and pubis, with associated separation of the pubic bones or of the sacro-iliac joints, constitute major and severe injuries. If the fracture is of the compression type with inward displacement of the fragments, adhesive traction should be applied to the leg of the side which is upwardly displaced. Twenty to 30 lb. of weight may be necessary, and should be maintained until the upward displacement is corrected. No binder or pelvic sling should be used for the side-

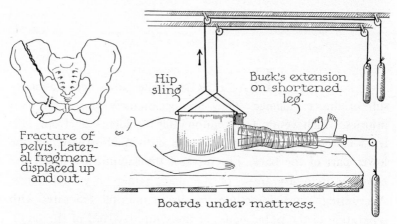

Hip sling

Buck's extension on shortened leg.

Fracture of pelvis. Lateral fragment displaced up and out.

Boards under mattress.

Fig. 217.—The pelvic sling is contraindicated when the fracture fragments are medially displaced.

to-side compression fractures. The patient should be made as comfortable as possible on a fracture bed which has arrangements for the use of the bedpan. For a woman in the child-bearing age, especial effort should be made to obtain anatomic restoration of all of the fragments involving the birth canal. When the fracture is produced by force directed anteroposteriorly against the pelvic bones, there may be wide separation at the symphysis, with displacement of sacro-iliac joints and lateral displacement of fracture fragments. If there is any asymmetry due to upward displacement, traction should be applied on the leg of

CHAPTER XXXII

The Ribs and Sternum

THE RIBS

FRACTURES of the ribs, often multiple, are common in adults and rare in children. They occur as a result of direct violence from a fall or a blow. They are sometimes complicated by separation of the costal cartilages. Costochondral dislocation without fracture may also occur. The patient may complain of pain in the chest, which is made worse by deep breathing or coughing. Though it rarely happens, the fractured rib may perforate the pleura and the lung, creating either emphysema or collapse of the lung.

Rib fractures can usually be demonstrated by roentgenogram. An incomplete fracture with no displacement may be difficult to identify, and separation of the costochondral junction without gross displacement cannot be diagnosed roentgenologically.

Fractures of the ribs without infection and without underlying pathology or injury to the lung usually heal whether treated or not. The patient can be made much more comfortable, however, by adhesive strapping or bandaging of the chest. When adhesive strapping is applied, it should extend from the nipple line on the side opposite the fracture to beyond the axillary border of the scapula on the back of the opposite side. Injection of 3 cc. of 1 per cent procaine into the hematoma at the site of each fracture before applying the adhesive strapping adds to the patient's comfort (Fig. 220).

Unless infection develops, emphysema can be ignored because the air is absorbed within a few days. Pneumothorax with dysp-

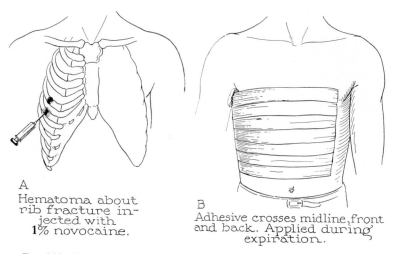

A

Hematoma about
rib fracture in-
jected with
1% novocaine.

B

Adhesive crosses midline, front
and back. Applied during
expiration.

Fig. 220.—Treatment of open fractures of the ribs by local infiltration of procaine and adequate adhesive dressing.

nea, due to collapse or compression of the lung, should be treated by repeated aspiration of the air. Treatment should be conservative in the presence of blood in the pleural cavity, which may be due to hemorrhage from an intercostal artery or from the lung. The bleeding may last for several days, and until it has presumably stopped no attempt should be made to remove the blood. In open fractures, all open breaks in the skin or lacerations of the chest wall should be débrided with the same care that is essential to obtaining good results in the treatment of any open fracture. The wound should be closed without burying any catgut, using only silk for the skin.

DOUBLE FRACTURES.—Occasionally, double fractures of all or nearly all of the ribs on one side will occur, with extensive crushing in of the chest wall. This injury is usually associated with partial or total atelectasis of the lung since on inspiration the

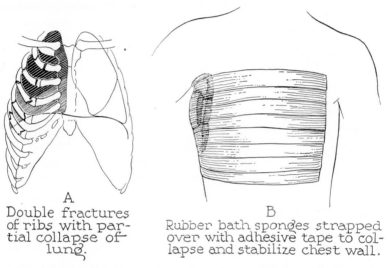

A
Double fractures of ribs with partial collapse of lung.

B
Rubber bath sponges strapped over with adhesive tape to collapse and stabilize chest wall.

FIG. 221.—Treatment of double fractures of the ribs and the associated collapse of the chest wall.

chest wall collapses and insufficient negative pressure can develop in the pleural cavity to expand the lung. The chest wall must be stabilized by a tight binding or strapping incorporating three or four rubber sponges over the site of the fractures (Fig. 221). This dressing should be replaced daily if necessary to maintain some rigidity of the thoracic cage and is not to be removed until there is clinical and roentgenographic evidence of union. This usually requires four weeks. The use of blow bottles will facilitate re-expansion of the lung.

THE STERNUM

The commonest cause of fracture of the sternum is a head-on collision of an automobile and another moving car or a stationary object, in which the driver is thrown forward with great force against the steering wheel. Another type of sternum fracture, seen much less frequently, is that sustained in conjunction with fractures of the vertebrae, produced by marked jackknife flexion of the trunk. A mechanic working underneath a car may suffer this combined injury if the jack turns over or breaks and the car comes down on his head and shoulders, doubling him sharply forward. A common location of this fracture is at the junction of the manubrium and gladiolus.

The sternum has a good deal of resilience. Cracks without complete separation of fragments may cause no serious disability. In complete fracture with separation, there may be difficulty in breathing and pain deep in the mediastinum as well as superficially. A lateral roentgenogram may show the fracture; the anteroposterior view is usually of little value. Fractures of the sternum are often associated with injuries of the ribs, clavicle, scapula or spine.

Open fracture of the sternum is especially dangerous because infection may develop, and if this happens, mediastinitis will almost certainly follow and is likely to be fatal. Treatment of fractures of the sternum without displacement consists of rest in bed. If the fracture is incomplete, adhesive strapping may be all that is required. For marked comminution with displacement of fragments, reduction should be attempted by hyperextending the spine, with the arms held overhead. A shoulder figure-of-eight plaster cast dressing, such as that used in fractures of the clavicle, carried down over the chest to the level of the tenth rib, affords a satisfactory method of immobilization. The patient should lie with a sandbag placed between the scapulae until the cast has firmly set and should be kept in bed until there is no longer pain on movement or deep breathing.

PART V

The Face and Skull

CHAPTER XXXIII

The Bones of the Face and Skull

THE more common fracture injuries of the face are those of the nasal bones, the malar zygomatic and the mandible. Dislocations in this region are exceedingly rare, with the exception of that of the temporomandibular joint.

THE FACE.—Fractures of the bones of the face are produced most often by direct violence, such as the impact of the face against the windshield of an automobile which has crashed head-on into another car or stationary object, throwing the occupants of the car forward. A blow from a fist or other blunt object may fracture the nose. These fractures are frequently open, or they may be associated with severe contusions or lacerations in other parts of the face, in which event these secondary injuries should receive priority in treatment. Scrupulous débridement should be performed as soon as possible after injury, followed by a plastic closure which will produce the least possible amount of scarring. Accurate reduction of all fractures of the bones of the face and jaw is important, because of the disfigurement which may result from malunion.

THE MANDIBLE.—This is the largest bone of the face. It is only through movement of the mandible at the temporomandibular joint that the mouth can be opened and closed. Biting and chewing are both made possible through the strength and integrity of this bone. A fracture of the mandible which fails to unite will seriously interfere with this function. Malunion of a fracture of the mandible will produce malocclusion of the teeth,

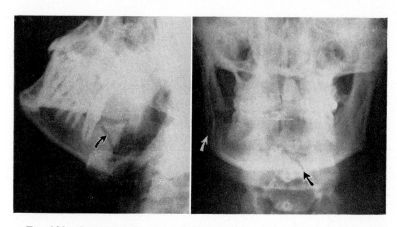

Fig. 222.—Segmental fracture of the mandible through the middle portion and through the region of the third molar. Moderate displacement was easily corrected and the position maintained with simple wire loops around the incisor teeth and small rubber band traction between the loops.

as well as asymmetry and disfigurement of the face. Fractures of the mandible most commonly occur in the portion nearest the chin, the ascending ramus or the neck of the condyle. They are occasionally bilateral.

A fracture of the mandible can be clinically diagnosed by the demonstration of false motion of the jaw and malocclusion of the teeth. Treatment should not be undertaken until a complete set of satisfactory roentgenograms has been obtained. They should be made from both sides and in the anteroposterior plane.

Uncomplicated fractures of the mandible should be reduced by gentle manipulation of the fragments and the position of normal occlusion maintained by rubber bands attached to wire loops around the teeth (Fig. 222). Wires of 26 or 28 gauge stainless steel are placed around two upper and two lower teeth on each side. Each wire is twisted tight and cut off to leave about ¼ in. of twist which is used as a hook for attachment of fixation. The canines are preferable for this purpose, but occasionally one must use the teeth of the fragments involved. The wires on the upper teeth are connected to the wires on the lower teeth by small rubber bands made by cutting narrow segments from a piece of latex tubing.

The teeth are carefully examined for uniform proper occlusion; this is specific for the particular patient undergoing treatment. It is therefore essential that the patient be questioned as to the nature of the occlusion before the accident.

Meticulous hygienic care is necessary during the period of immobilization of the jaw. The teeth, wires and rubber bands must be brushed after each meal with warm water. The inside of the mouth is rinsed repeatedly with warm water or a commercial mouth wash. The patient must not try to open the mouth, and an adequate liquid diet is prescribed. Soft food can be ingested if some teeth are missing.

The teeth are released after four weeks, although roentgenograms will not show bony union for several months. Comminuted fractures of the mandible must be immobilized for six to eight weeks.

Open reduction and internal fixation by wiring the fragments together may be necessary if the patient is edentulous. Occasionally, after reduction or in fractures without displacement, artificial dentures can be used as internal splints, with the mouth bandaged closed with an elastic bandage. The incision for open reduction is placed beneath the mandible for the optimal cosmetic result.

Patients with a posteriorly displaced midfragment of the mandible require special consideration. It is necessary to bring the fragment forward to align it properly with the other portions of the mandible and to restore normal occlusion. The reduction is usually accomplished by digital manipulation. Wire loops are then placed around the teeth as for a closed fracture, and the teeth of the loose fragment are fixed in proper occlusion to a bridge of German silver that spans the fragment from sound teeth to sound teeth.

Complications of fractures of the jaw, other than those of malunion with malocclusion, may include infection. Most fractures of the body of the jaw bone break through the mucous membrane lining the mouth. If particles of food can be kept out of the compound wound, primary healing may be expected. The laceration should be closed with a few sutures. A tooth in the line of fracture is ordinarily extracted in order to prevent the formation of an abscess. Caution must be exercised when the fracture is at the angle of the jaw. If the second or third molar is extracted, the bone fragment may be displaced by muscle pull. It is preferable to leave these teeth in place, at least until a local complication makes extraction imperative.

Osteomyelitis following an open fracture should be treated by drainage through the skin overlying the bone at the site of the infection. In placing the incision, consideration should be given to the cosmetic effect and an attempt made to provide the drainage medial to the lower border of the mandible where the scar will be less obvious.

Ununited fractures of the jaw, without infection, or after the infection has been healed for several months, may be treated successfully by a bone graft obtained from the tibia or ilium and inlaid across the fracture line. If a full thickness portion of the mandible has been lost through sequestration, a graft which accurately matches the defect in the bone may be removed from the crest of the ilium and placed in the defect with the ends overlapping each fragment of the jaw. Fractures which have healed with extreme malunion and malocclusion are not suitable for re-fracture in an attempt to obtain better position. It may be advisable to remove the teeth and have them replaced with a denture. Occasionally osteotomy of the ascending ramus and correction of mandibular protrusion or retraction are necessary.

DISLOCATION OF THE TEMPOROMANDIBULAR JOINT.—This may occur during the act of yawning, during an attempt to bite into an apple or orange or as a result of direct violence, and may be associated with fracture. Simple dislocation is recognized by the fact that the jaw is held open and swallowing is difficult. It is impossible for the patient to close the jaw. If the accident has occurred only a few minutes prior to examination, there will be pain and spasm of the pterygoid muscle. Palpation reveals dislocation of the mandibular head.

Reduction of dislocation of the temporomandibular articulation is relatively easy. The surgeon should carefully wrap his thumbs with cotton or a towel, place them in the mouth and press downward on the angles of the jaws at the same time that his fingers are raising the chin. The reduction occurs with a sharp snap, and there is simultaneously a sudden contraction of the muscles of mastication. If the thumbs have not been protected, they may be severely lacerated by the patient's teeth. Following a single unilateral dislocation, no bandage or any type of immobilization is necessary. If the dislocation was bilateral, a firm bandage should be wrapped from beneath the chin around the parietal bone.

FRACTURE-DISLOCATIONS.—Open operation may be required to reduce the dislocation, followed by treatment of the fracture, as described for the treatment of a closed fracture.

THE ZYGOMA.—This bone shapes the contour of the cheek. Injuries occur as a result of a direct blow. The depression is usually obvious immediately, but it may be obscured later by swelling of the soft parts. The depression is difficult to demonstrate in the roentgenogram, but it may be noted on careful palpation. Distortion of the orbit may produce diplopia. The fracture is most successfully treated by inserting a long periosteal elevator through a short incision made in the edge of the hairline just in front of the ear. The fractured portion of the zygoma may then be elevated until the flattening of this portion of the face is no longer present. Rarely is additional treatment necessary.

THE MAXILLA.—Closed fractures of the maxilla without displacement are treated by holding the teeth aligned with wire loops and rubber bands as described for fractures of the mandible.

If the fracture is bilateral and one can move the patient's face from side to side while grasping the nose, it is necessary to obtain compression by means of a skull cap connected by rubber bands to a plaster mold under the chin. An ordinary surgeon's cap can be used and a chin piece made by molding a slab of plaster over a piece of felt fitted to the chin with a strip of muslin interposed between the felt and plaster.

The wire bands are attached to the side margins of the cap and the ends of the muslin. If the bite is poor, the teeth are fixed with wires and bands in proper occlusion. Centrally displaced fragments are brought forward and attached to a bar of half round of German silver wire. Immobilization is continued for six weeks, although union is not complete for three to six months.

The third type of fracture of the maxilla involves the floor of the orbit and produces diplopia. Treatment consists of making an incision in the lower lid over the fracture and elevation of the fragments under direct vision by means of a urethral sound passed into the antrum. The fragments are maintained in position by $1/2$ in. petrolatum gauze packed into the antrum. The end of the pack is pulled out through the nose. It may be necessary to perforate the nasal wall beneath the turbinate to accomplish this treatment. In some cases the fragments of the malar bone must be wired together while the fracture is exposed in order to maintain the reduction. Antibiotics are given in adequate doses to guard against infection. If the temperature remains elevated to 101 or 102 degrees for two or three days, it is necessary to remove the pack; otherwise, the pack is not removed for 10 to 14 days.

Special skill is required in the treatment of fractures of the

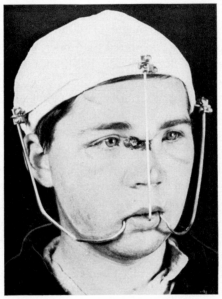

Fig. 223.—Fracture of the maxillae with displacement, corrected by a plaster skull cap and wires attached to a prosthesis which fits the contour of the hard palate.

maxillary bone, and it is best performed by those with specialized training.

THE NASAL BONES.—Fractures of the nasal bones may be the result of lateral or of vertical blows, with corresponding types of fracture displacements. These fractures are too often neglected, and many persons go through life with inferiority complexes caused by crooked noses which followed injuries sustained during childhood or adolescence. All displacements of fractures of the nasal bones should be corrected under either local or general anesthesia. Small forceps may be introduced through the nostril until they lie beneath the nasal crest. The depressed fragments may then be gently elevated, while the outside contour of the nose is molded by the thumb and fingers of the operator's left hand. A plastic splint may be molded over the nose to hold alignment of the nasal bridge, while a rubber sponge is maintained inside the nose. Single or double wire splints of the Watson-Williams type, protected by rubber, are efficient in keeping the fragments elevated into position and cause relatively little discomfort.

FRACTURES OF THE BONES OF THE CALVARIUM.—These present almost no problem from the standpoint of treatment. Much ado is made over the fact that the roentgenogram shows fractures in the bones of the skull, but such injuries are of far less significance than is the question of the extent of damage to the brain which often accompanies them. Furthermore, concussion of the brain or more serious brain injury may occur when there is no fracture of the skull. *Every injury to the head must be considered as possibly related to a brain injury, whether the skull is fractured or not.*

HEAD INJURIES.—Carefully planned management of head injuries, whether or not there is a fracture of the calvarium, will reduce the mortality rate by 25 to 50 per cent. The most dangerous period is the first six hours. The following outline of treatment is recommended.

1. Transfer the patient from stretcher to bed. Place him between blankets and apply heat.
2. Make a roentgen examination of every head injury, *but not until evidence of cerebral shock has subsided.*
3. Suture scalp wounds.
4. Do not transfer the patient from one ward to another or to another hospital.

5. Avoid oversedation. Do not give morphine; morphine masks the picture and adds to respiratory depression.

6. Examine the eyegrounds for evidence of edema.

7. Stimulate if necessary, but do not depend on stimulants and sedation as the sole treatment.

8. Make a spinal puncture if the patient becomes increasingly stuporous.

9. Intravenous administration of sucrose, 50 cc. of 50 per cent solution, is the best means of restoring blood volume in shock. An additional 200–300 cc. of isotonic sodium chloride should be used if indicated. Overcoming the shock, not the dehydration, is the sole purpose here.

10. Blood plasma or blood transfusion should be given if shock is profound or if there is hemorrhage from associated injuries.

11. Oxygen therapy will tide many a patient over this dangerous period.

12. Postural drainage or the use of an aspirator is always indicated when the air passages are obstructed.

13. Antitetanus, antigas and other prophylactic serums may contribute additional insult. Their administration should be delayed at least six hours after injury.

14. Watch and record the pulse, respiratory rate and blood pressure every 30 minutes to one hour and the temperature every one to two hours; observe changes in the pupils and reflexes.

BASAL SKULL FRACTURES.—Fractures of the vault of the calvarium are less likely to be associated with intracranial trauma than are fractures at the base of the skull. Symptoms of basal skull fracture may include bleeding from the ears or nose and relatively minor local evidence of trauma. There may be more damage to the brain than with multiple fractures of the vault of the skull, which result from more severe violence. If the patient survives the injury to the brain, the fracture of the skull will heal without manipulation or immobilization.

Severely depressed fractures of the skull may carry a portion of the bone deep into the brain tissue, requiring open operation and elevation of the depressed fragments. Symptoms of acute intracranial pressure are indications for decompression operations. They not only relieve the pressure, but permit inspection of major brain surfaces and of the arteries and veins which may have been damaged, so that hemorrhage may be controlled by ligation.

Open fractures of the skull which are associated with laceration of the scalp (or with involvement of the sinuses, an orbit or the inner ear) may lead to infection unless they are dealt with adequately. When the open fracture includes laceration of the scalp, careful cleansing, débridement and suture should be carried out as soon as treatment for shock has been instituted.

Index

NOTE.—An asterisk (*) following a page number indicates an illustration.